Respiratory
Nuts and Bolts

by
Michael J. Fischer, RRT

Contents

1 Respiratory Review 1

2 Assessment Skills 5

3 Respiratory Disease 17

4 Oxygen and Oxygen Delivery 30

5 Respiratory Therapy Treatments. 50

6 Respiratory Failure and Airway Management. 67

7 Introduction to Mechanical Ventilation 84

8 Modes of Mechanical Ventilation 94

9 Arterial Blood Gases 119

Introduction

PROFESSIONAL DEVELOPMENT IS THE PROCESS OF ACQUIRING THE knowledge and skills needed to be proficient in a chosen career field. The first component of professional development is typically a good, scholastic education consisting of high school and often times collegiate-level classes. The field you choose to practice in will determine how much education is required to gain an entry-level position into the workforce.

The second phase of professional development occurs when you have obtained your entry-level position and have arrived for your first day of work. This phase is often referred to as on-the-job training.

Many impromptu discussions have been held around the water cooler regarding how best to prepare someone for the workforce. Some argue that a well-rounded education is the cornerstone of proficiency in the workplace. Others claim that it isn't until someone experiences the "real" world before they find out what they are made of. They will make a case that once you are out of school, the real education begins.

Many textbooks are thrust upon you at the collegiate level. Most textbooks are similar in how they are constructed. Oh sure, the topic changes from book to book, but the overall way the book is laid out is pretty much the same. This book is different.

The on-the-job training approach is designed to combine both levels of professional development into one. It is written as if you just showed up for your first day of work. The content is the content you would be receiving while on the job. This approach takes out much of the "fluff," which the typical textbook covers, and provides you with the substance that employers want you to know.

In no way am I telling you that your other textbooks are not a valuable resource, nor will this book be a substitution to the collegiate textbooks you already have or will obtain. This book will be an invaluable tool to you because, as you read through, you will get a true understanding of what a typical workday in your new career may look like. You will get a sense of what will be expected from you and what you can expect from the profession you work in.

RESPIRATORY NUTS AND BOLTS: is designed to be a small part of your on-the-job training as you enter the medical field. As a respiratory therapist of many years (no, I'm not going to tell you how long I've been at this. . .just let the gray hairs be a guide), I have been asked repeatedly to give certain classes about respiratory to non-respiratory personnel as they begin their medical careers. This is needed as some of the respiratory responsibilities do cross over to other professions. It all depends on the facility in which you work, but those responsibilities that cross over will be greater in some places than in others.

Not every facility will provide you with the best "cross-training" program, so instead of waiting for the reliability of that first job's training session, this book is intended to give you a head start in the knowledge that you will need to have in this field.

Through my years of working as a respiratory therapist, I have been able to develop quite an extensive amount of training for mainly nurses and resident physicians. I am taking all of the classes I teach on a regular basis and putting them in this book for you.

You will probably not need to know every topic that I cover. This will be dependent on where in the hospital you choose to work. Time can be saved if you skip to the chapters that pertain to your particular interest. The other chapters might be valuable to you later down the road if you choose to change your career path in the medical field.

It is my hope that you find this book to be a valuable resource to your library while you advance in your career of choice.

1

Respiratory Review

My INTENTION IN THIS CHAPTER IS TO GIVE YOU A REVIEW OF some of the important aspects of the respiratory system. I could certainly spend a great deal of time going into depth on many of these topics, but that would be counter intuitive to what I am trying to achieve, which is a quick and basic guideline. I feel there are highlights that should be covered, items of importance that will surface later in this text.

Anatomy and Physiology

The structures of the respiratory system and how they work are vast and complex. There are certain key points I want you to think about as we learn how to care for our pulmonary patient.

The primary function of the respiratory system is to provide oxygen to the tissues of the body and to eliminate carbon dioxide. It is absolutely vital that we always keep this primary function in mind. Everything we do for our patient is centered on this premise. Its definition is quite simple, but its application can get very complicated.

EXTERNAL RESPIRATION: is the process of bringing oxygen from the atmosphere into the lungs, and then through the process of diffusion, having that oxygen cross over from the alveoli into the blood stream. Subsequently, this process also includes carbon dioxide diffusing from the blood stream into the alveolus of the lung and then out into the atmosphere.

INTERNAL RESPIRATION: is the process of gas exchange between the blood and the tissues. Again, oxygen leaves the blood and enters the tissues as the carbon dioxide exits the tissues and accesses the bloodstream. You may also hear this referred to as *cellular respiration*.

Many problems can occur to prevent a patient's adequate gas exchange. The barrier can be related to an external respiratory problem, such as an obstructed airway. At other times, it can be an internal respiratory problem, such as in cyanide toxicity. When our patient is having issues, either from poor oxygenation or an elevated carbon dioxide level, we must attempt to identify where the problem lies. There are different strategies for correcting each set of problems, which I will discuss later.

THE UPPER AIRWAYS: again, there are many components to the upper airways, but what I want to focus on is their function. The main function, of course, is to act as a conduit for air to travel from the atmosphere to the lower airways. However, along this course, the upper airways provide some extremely vital functions for the health and well-being of our lungs and body as a whole: they *heat, humidify,* and *filter* the inspired air.

Yes, the upper airways do even more than this. These three functions, however, are key when it comes to some of the *modalities* we will use later to treat our patient.

THE MUSCLES OF RESPIRATION: The primary muscles of respiration are the *diaphragm* and the *intercostals*. There are many other smaller/accessory muscles of ventilation that I won't bore you with right now. The important point to take away from here is in regard to the assessment of our patient. During normal respiration, the *diaphragm* and the *intercostals* work quietly while doing their job. In viewing this type of patient, you will note that there is very little chest rise or fall. When someone is struggling to breathe, often times they will enlist the help of the accessory muscles. You may notice the shoulders rising and falling, which are known as *intercostal retractions*.

THE LOBES OF THE LUNGS: The right lung has three lobes (upper, middle, and lower), while the left has two lobes (upper and lower).

THE ALVEOLAR-CAPILLARY MEMBRANE (AKA A-C MEMBRANE OR BLOOD-GAS BARRIER): This membrane separates the alveoli from the bloodstream. It is the area where gas exchange takes place. Understanding the concept of gas exchange can help us when trying to correct problems via mechanical ventilation.

Mechanics of Ventilation

In a nutshell, this is the process of breathing. We breathe in; we breathe out. I know, I'm a genius, right? As I stated when I mentioned the primary function of respiration, the concept is easy, but the process can be difficult. It is important that you understand certain terminology as we proceed with this text.

TIDAL VOLUME: This is the amount of air, usually measured in ml, that moves in and out of the lungs in a given breath. The purpose of this tidal volume breath is to move oxygen into the body and carbon dioxide out of the body. The size of the tidal volume breath will vary, depending on the changing needs of the body. While during exercise, for example, the tidal volume breaths will increase to keep up with the metabolic demands of the body.

RESPIRATORY RATE: The number of breaths a person takes in a given minute. Again, this value will change depending on the demands of the body.

MINUTE VENTILATION: This is how much air is moving in and out of the lungs in a given minute, usually measured in ml. Mathematically speaking, it is the respiratory rate multiplied by the tidal volume.

$\dot{V} = V_T \times f$
$\dot{v}$ = Minute Ventilation
V_T = Tidal Volume
f = Frequency

Since the purpose of respiration or ventilation is basically the process of gas exchange, it is considered effective when CO_2 levels remain within normal limits. The normal limit is 35-45 mm Hg. This allows the blood pH to stay within normal limits of 7.35 to 7.45 mm Hg as well. I will be covering more about pH and CO_2 levels later under the topic of blood gases.

HYPOVENTILATION: This is a condition in which ventilation is below normal. It causes a rise in the CO_2, thus causing a drop in the blood pH.

HYPERVENTILATION: This is a condition in which ventilation is above normal. It causes a drop in the CO_2, thus causing a rise in the blood pH.

2

Assessment Skills

As you enter any patient care area in one of today's modern hospitals, it is plain to see how technology has invaded the healthcare industry: electronic/computerized monitoring is now available, wireless cardiac monitoring exists, microchip technology drives ventilators, and new technology has made lab results quicker and more accurate than ever before.

Along with these new technologies comes a new set of problems, and these problems must be addressed. The first, main problem is that the caregiver may develop a *dependence* on these new technologies even though we are taught to "treat the *patient*, not the monitor." Monitors can give erroneous results, lab machines can falter and provide poor data, and power failure can lead to interruptions, causing the hospital or clinic to go into what are called "downtime" procedures.

My point is this: *no amount of technology can replace good patient assessment skills.* Our ability to assess a patient is the most vital function that we can bring to the workplace. When a monitor says our patient's heart rhythm is flat-lined, we don't immediately code the patient. We *look* at the patient and *assess* if the monitor is correct (or at least I hope we do).

My brother has been a musician for 40 years now, and he is proficient in many instruments. Despite all of his talent and skills, you can still catch him playing the basic musical scales on any given day. He tells me this is fundamental. Once you can play the scales to perfection, you are then ready to learn how to string some notes together, using those fundamental scales as your "guides."

We need to look at our assessment skills as the "musical scales" of our profession. We are not ready to take the first step toward treating a patient until we can properly assess them, or in other words, until we have mastered the basic fundamentals of patient assessment.

The purpose of this chapter is to lay down the fundamental foundations of patient assessment in hopes that you will become more proficient in giving the most effective respiratory assessments of your future patients.

General Inspection

Upon entering the patient's room, you must process a lot of information rather quickly. Once you have entered, make *eye contact* with the patient while *taking note* of others in the room. Keep your senses sharp and pay close attention to the mood in the room. If it appears somber, you will approach the situation differently than perhaps a room where people are talking and laughing. You never know when a patient may have received some difficult information, and you want to be empathetic to whatever situation you have entered into.

While still maintaining eye contact with your patient, let them know who you are. State your first name, your job title, and the reason for your visit. For security reasons, many healthcare workers do not give their first and last name. You may want to ask the patient at this time how they are feeling and how their breathing is today.

As I mentioned above, a lot of things will happen fairly quickly, and it is vital for you to pay close attention to detail as your assessment of the patient has begun. Assessment of the patient involves most *all* of your senses. You need to communicate effectively, both verbally and non-verbally. You need to listen carefully to what the patient has to say as well as to those in the room who know the patient. Sometimes the patient is unable to provide every detail that we would like, perhaps due to the medications they are on, the overall mental status, or just the stress that they may be under at that point.

Pay attention to the environment and ask the patient if they are comfortable or if they are too warm or too cold. Meanwhile, look over your patient quickly from head to toe to get an initial "feel" of how they present themselves. If they appear to be distressed or are exhibiting any signs of a life-threatening condition, call for assistance immediately and perform any supportive measures within your scope of practice while waiting for help. If the patient's mental status is altered from what was reported or what you have seen previously, you will want to get immediate assistance before continuing on with your assessment. One of the primary ways to assess for level of consciousness is by asking the patient who they are, where they are, and what time it is.

If none of the above conditions are present and the patient appears to be within their "baseline" status, then proceed with your assessment.

Observe for symptoms such as:

Dyspnea: This is not a breathing pattern, but it *is* a symptom. We define it as shortness of breath. We cannot depend on our senses to determine if a patient is short of breath, as it is subjective, so a more accurate definition of dyspnea is *what the patient perceives* as shortness of breath.

COUGH: Does the patient have a persistent cough? How does it sound? Is it productive? How long have they had it?

SECRETIONS: Does the patient have secretions? If so, do the secretions have an odor and/or color? What is the amount of the secretions? Are they thick or thin? Is there blood present?

PAIN: Does it hurt the patient to breathe or cough? Do they have chest pain? If they do have chest pain, what is it like?

EDEMA: I know we are trained to look for edema primarily in the extremities. What we need to keep in mind is that if there is noticeable edema in the extremities, there is a good chance that some form of pulmonary edema is occurring as well. It is important to keep an adequate record of the patient's fluid intake and output to determine if there is a "fluid overload" problem. If a patient is experiencing decreased oxygen levels and increased work of breathing, it may simply be a matter of giving a diuretic such as Lasix rather than administering a medication such as Albuterol via a handheld nebulizer.

Vital Signs

I am not going to go into detail on all of the vital signs. Instead I'm just going to go over the normal values. I will go into detail on oxygen saturation as I feel that is a vital sign which is commonly misunderstood.

Heart rate:

Newborn	1-12 months	1-2 years	2-6 years	6-12 years	13-adult
120-160	80-140	80-130	75-120	75-110	60-100

Blood pressure:

Newborn	1-12 months	1-2 years	2-6 years	6-12 years	13-adult
120-160	80-140	80-130	75-120	75-110	60-100

Respiratory rate:

Newborns	Less than 1 year	1-3 years	3-6 years	6-12 years	12-adult
30-40	30-40	23-35	20-30	18-26	12-20

OXYGEN SATURATION: basically measures the amount of hemoglobin binding sites that are occupied by oxygen. We measure this as a percentage, and the normal value is usually between 95% and 100%. In some conditions, such as patients with Chronic Obstructive Pulmonary Disease (COPD), the normal values may be lower. The measurement is taken with the use of a pulse oximeter. A pulse oximeter is a probe that is usually placed on the finger and emits two wavelengths of light (650nm and 805nm), which are absorbed by the hemoglobin molecules. The more saturated the hemoglobin molecules are with a gas, such as oxygen, the more this light will be absorbed. The probe then calculates the amount of light absorbed and reads it as a percentage on its screen.

It is important to understand that this measurement is not always correct. False readings can occur. If the patient has on fake nails or a dark-colored nail polish, both of these can prevent the light from penetrating the skin and thus give a false, low reading. Also, if the skin is not adequately perfused, an adequate reading may be hard to obtain. If the hands are cold to the touch, it might be an indication that perfusion is not adequate. If the reading is alarmingly low, always be sure to look at your patient. An extremely low saturation reading will usually be accompanied by a patient who is short of breath, cyanotic, or ashen in appearance. If the patient feels fine and their color is healthy, don't be overly alarmed over your saturation reading. Remember the old adage, "treat the *patient*, not the monitor." Monitors *do* have a tendency to malfunction.

Chest Assessment

The chest assessment is a major part of the overall respiratory assessment of the patient and includes the following aspects:

1. Inspection
2. Palpation
3. Percussion
4. Auscultation

Inspection:

Visualize the chest as the patient breathes. Are both the left and right side of the chest rising equally? An unequal rise could be an indication of a problem such as a pneumothorax.

Next, assess the breathing pattern. If you have spent any amount of time in the medical field, especially if that time has been served in a Critical Care Unit, then you know by now that our patients will exhibit quite a variety of different breathing patterns. I have listed the major types of patterns in Box 1-1.

How do we treat these patterns? We don't typically just treat the patterns as much as we treat the other symptoms associated with the pattern. If the respiratory pattern, along with its associated symptoms, demonstrates that the patient cannot sustain adequate ventilation and oxygenation, then they may be placed on non-invasive ventilation or intubated. Sometimes supplemental oxygen is all that is required.

Box 1-1

Breathing Pattern	Definition	Causes
Apnea	A period in which no breathing is occurring.	Overdose, trauma, and airway obstruction.
Apneustic	Deep, gasping inspiration with a pause at the end of inspiration, followed by a short expiratory period.	Neurological damage usually caused by trauma or stroke.
Biot's	Quick, shallow inspirations followed by periods of apnea.	Neurological damage usually caused by trauma or stroke.
Cheyne-Stokes	Progressively faster and deeper breathing followed by a gradual decrease, leading to a period of apnea.	Heart failure, stroke, and sleep apnea.
Kussmaul's	Deep and labored breathing pattern.	Diabetic keto-acidosis, uremia, peritonitis, and pneumonia.
Paradoxical	Portion or all of the chest wall moves in with inhalation and out with exhalation.	Chest trauma and flail chest.

Palpation:

Palpation is the act of feeling with the hand or fingers. Some data we can collect via the process of palpation is as follows:

VOCAL FREMITUS: Fremitus is defined as a vibration. Thus, vocal fremitus while palpating the chest means that you feel a vibration on the chest wall as the patient speaks. The best way to test for vocal fremitus is to have the patient repeat the word "ninety-nine" as you place your hands on the chest. If you feel fremitus, this is a sign of a consolidation, or fluid in the lungs. I have also felt this on intubated patients on occasion. As the air leaves the patient, I can sometimes feel fremitus on the chest wall and even the respiratory circuit as well.

SUBCUTANEOUS AIR: This phenomenon occurs when air escapes the lungs in the subcutaneous space. It often happens with some form of chest trauma, such as a gunshot wound or rib fractures. It is characterized by a crackling feel or sensation to the skin and is usually felt in the chest, neck, or face regions. You will often times hear that crackling feel referred to as "Rice Krispies."

Percussion:

I am not going to spend a lot of time on this skill as it takes a great deal of experience, and in my opinion, can lead to a mis-diagnosis unless performed by someone such as a pulmonologist or ICU attending physician who has a vast amount of experience performing this technique. It is basically the process of tapping along the surface of the chest wall. Based on the sound heard with the tapping, the physician can get an idea of the underlying structures; for example, if they are fluid-filled or air-filled.

Auscultation:

This is the process of listening to the internal sounds of the body. In our case, we will be discussing the internal sounds produced by the lungs. The process of auscultation is performed with the use of a stethoscope. Note that the medical community uses a variety of breath sound descriptions, but there has not been a standardized or unified set of terminology, which makes describing the sounds difficult. I will attempt to use the most common descriptions, but bear in mind that, depending on where you work, you might hear some terms used that I have not covered. Also keep in mind that no amount of description can replace the actual hearing of the sounds. It takes a great deal of time to gain enough experience, which will help you truly recognize the various lung sounds and identify their causes.

Breath Sounds

NORMAL BREATH SOUNDS: basically sound like wind or air being delivered over a large pipe. Depending on where you place your stethoscope, the sounds you hear will be lower or higher-pitched in sound due to the various sizes of the airways.

TRACHEAL BREATH SOUNDS: for example, are heard when listening over the trachea, which is a relatively large "pipe." The sound will be lower-pitched.

BRONCHIAL BREATH SOUNDS: are heard primarily over the upper-third of the anterior part of the chest. The air passing through this portion of your lung space is loud and a little higher-pitched than tracheal breath sounds as the airways are now smaller in diameter.

VESICULAR BREATH SOUNDS: are more "soft and blowing" and are heard throughout most of the lung fields. They are heard throughout expiration and start to fade out about a third of the way through inspiration.

CRACKLES: are a kind of "popping" sound. Some say they sound like Rice Krispies in milk or Velcro being pulled away. This sound is representative of smaller airways "popping open." The small airways have somehow become obstructed and completely closed off during the expiratory phase, and it is because of this closing that they take more effort to reopen, thus the "popping" sound. This is treated either with bronchodilators or through inspiratory maneuvers that help to recruit (open) the alveoli, such as incentive spirometers or Intermittent Positive Pressure Breathing (IPPB). Another term for crackles that you may hear is "rales."

RHONCHI: sounds a bit like snoring. It is a more coarse sound that is usually caused by an obstruction in the large airways. This also may occur when loose secretions are present in the airways. As the air moves past these secretions, it causes them to move and rattle. Because rhonchi resemble snoring, it is important to make sure that it is in fact *not* snoring. If a patient is asleep and snoring, the snoring sound may resonate to the lower airways, giving the appearance that the sound is actually being generated from the lungs rather than the upper airway. This can result in a misdiagnosis. Any maneuver that helps the patient have a more productive cough can help this problem. If the patient is unable to produce an effective cough, suctioning the airway may be needed.

WHEEZES: sound like a high-pitched whistling and are more commonly heard during inspiration. This is the result of a narrowing of the airways, such as during an asthma attack, and can be treated by the use of a bronchodilator (more on that later). Wheezes are not always high-pitched in nature; they can also be a lower pitch, which is more commonly heard over the larger airways during constriction.

STRIDOR: is a more severe-sounding wheeze that primarily affects the upper airway. It is usually audible without a stethoscope, and once you have heard it, you will not forget what it sounds like. It typically indicates a swelling of the upper airway and can be found in patients who have epiglottitis, a foreign body aspiration (choking), or thermal injury resulting from a household fire. This is typically treated with a cool mist aerosol or having the patient breathe into a nebulizer containing racemic epinephrine.

PLEURAL FRICTION RUBS: sound like a "creaking" or "squeaking" sound. The pleural linings rubbing together cause these, such as in the case with pleurisy. If you are unsure of what you are hearing, your patient should give it away as it is usually quite painful for the patient to breathe under such a condition.

DIMINISHED OR ABSENT BREATH SOUNDS: occur when the flow of air is reduced or completely stopped due to some sort of obstruction. This could be due to a mucus plug, a reduction in the size of the airway caused by bronchoconstriction, or by obesity. When there is more tissue to listen through to hear the breath sounds, it could give the appearance of diminished or absent breath sounds when the real problem is that you are simply trying to pick up the breath sounds through too much tissue.

The quality of the stethoscope could also be a problem. Patients in isolation rooms are typically required to have a dedicated stethoscope for their room. Disposable stethoscopes provided by the facility are often used. These stethoscopes are not as high in quality as many that could be purchased through a variety of vendors, and thus the use of these stethoscopes could also give the false impression of diminished breath sounds.

Many times I am asked to listen to breath sounds from someone who is not quite sure what they have heard. Sometimes noises are heard that do not fit any of the descriptions listed above. The two things I always tell people are this: first, as is mentioned above, there is no universally-accepted standard of definitions to describe breath sounds, so don't get too hung up on it; second, just describe what you hear. I have seen and heard people describe breath sounds as "wet rales," "wet rhonchi," "squeaky," etc. Here are some phrases that I have heard to describe breath sounds, none of which I would use in my documentation: "sounds like a washing machine," "sounds like they are breathing through pond water," or my all-time favorite, "sounds like crap." Yes, sometimes our medical jargon is a little loose.

3

Respiratory Disease

ONCE AGAIN, I FIND MYSELF AT A CROSSROADS, DECIDING WHAT to discuss and what to eliminate. When it comes to airway disease, there are scores of books and literature available. I want to focus on the two biggest respiratory disease processes that we manage on a regular basis: COPD and asthma. Again, I could bore you to death with all the intricacies involved here, but instead I want to give a brief overview. I wish to cover things I think you really need to know and focus on, eliminate some myths, and teach you how to perform certain tasks and functions which I have seen done wrong on many an occasion.

Chronic Obstructive Pulmonary Disease (COPD)

As its name suggests, this is an obstructive disease process of the lungs, resulting in the restriction of airflow. Emphysema and chronic bronchitis are the two most common conditions that make up COPD:

- **Emphysema:** Characterized by abnormal and permanent enlargement of the airspaces beyond the terminal bronchiole. Over time, it destroys the walls of the airspaces.

17

- **Chronic bronchitis:** Defined as having a chronic, productive cough for at least three months of the year for two consecutive years.

Signs and symptoms include:

- Chronic cough
- Sputum production
- Wheezing
- Shortness of breath
- Chronic fatigue
- Anxiety

Diagnosis of COPD can be complicated. There is no one, true test to determine this disease. It is a culmination of the patient's history, signs and symptoms, and a few tests. Some tests that can provide valuable information are that of a chest x-ray and a pulmonary function test.

I have been in this profession for a long time now, and one thing I can say for certain is that if you have a patient who smokes, that does not mean they have COPD. I can't tell you how many times we have had a patient admitted, already intubated and unable to speak, and the limited history includes the fact that he/she is or was a heavy smoker. Many of these patients have rarely (if ever) seen a doctor, so establishing a "baseline" is difficult. Yet given this limited information, one of the most common lines I hear is, "They are a smoker, and probably have COPD, so their baseline pulmonary status probably isn't very good." If I had a dollar for every time I've heard that, I'd own my own private island somewhere.

As I've said, I've been at this a while. I've also seen many patients who have smoked heavily since they were in diapers. Now they are 90, have never been sick, have never been short of breath, and can run a marathon. . .backwards!! I've also seen patients in their 20s, who have only smoked for a short while, have significant COPD at such an early age, and they can't even spell "marathon" without collapsing.

My point is this: it is a colossal mistake to blatantly diagnose someone with such a horrendous disease while only having limited information, and it has *got* to *stop*. When we do this, patients get mistreated and outcomes suffer.

Another "common" characteristic of COPD patients is that they may have a chronically-high CO_2 level in their blood. It's O.K. They are used to this as it is a chronic condition, and the body adjusts. This is all part of the obstructive process of the disease. As it progresses, it gets harder and harder for the patient to exhale effectively. Also, because of the ineffectiveness of the patient's lungs, they may suffer from a chronically-low oxygen level. Many COPD patients need to wear oxygen on a regular basis.

This leads to another common problem which I witness on a regular basis. When we have a COPD patient, a common line I hear is this, "Well, they have COPD, so they probably live with a CO_2 level around 60 and an O_2 level of around 60 as well." This is also called the 60/60 Club. Although it may be true for some of the COPD population, it is certainly not indicative of the entire population. Most of these problems actually occur in the late stages of COPD. So again, unless we know what the true "baseline" status of the patient is, we must be careful not to assume that every COPD patient falls into this classification.

The last, big problem I want to cover when caring for the COPD patient is that of the Hypoxic Drive Theory. Clinicians are quick to say, "Don't give this patient too much oxygen, or you'll knock out the hypoxic drive." This topic can get extensive, so let me just leave you with this: it is called a theory for a reason. Some believe in it 100%, others don't believe in it at all. In my opinion, it affects a very small population of COPD patients. I have seen it maybe 5 times in my career. An article I once read states that it doesn't matter. If the patient needs oxygen, they need oxygen. Most of us work in a controlled environment; if we give too much oxygen and the patient stops breathing, we can fix this by intubating them. If we don't give enough oxygen and the patient suffers hypoxic tissue damage, we can't reverse this. A favorite quote I once read goes:

"Hypoxia kills; hypercapnia happens."
—Dr. Busko

Busko.   http://www.learnmoresavelives.com/blog/copd-and-myth-hypoxic-drive-mediated-sudden-hyperoxic-death-oh-my (Accessed 11/05/09)

Exacerbation of COPD:

This is simply a worsening of the symptoms. The worsening can be anywhere from mild to severe. It is important, especially for the COPD patients themselves, to recognize when an exacerbation process has begun. It does not take long for COPD to digress to a life-threatening condition, thus all cases of exacerbation must be treated severely and aggressively. A patient who is familiar with their home regiment and symptoms may be able to avoid seeking medical assistance. However, they should always be able to recognize when the condition is getting out of their control and seek medical help before it is too late.

Treating COPD:

COPD causes irreversible damage to the airways, so it is important to begin treatment right away in order to try and slow down the damaging effects. First and foremost, it is imperative to remove oneself from the environment that has caused the disease. In most cases, the cause of COPD is from smoking, thus enrolling in a qualified smoking cessation program is of the utmost importance. The patient may be prescribed a host of available medications. Again, the medications prescribed depend on the severity of the patient's condition and symptoms. Here are a few common medications, which I will cover more on later:

<u>Bronchodilators</u>	<u>Corticosteroids</u>
Albuterol	Flovent
Atrovent	Solumedrol
Combivent	Prednisone
Spiriva	Advair
Terbutaline	Beclomethasone
Theophylline	Budesonide
Xopenex	Flunisolide
Formoterol	Mometasone
Salmeterol	Triamcinolone

Some patients will require the use of supplemental oxygen, which may only be needed during an exacerbation episode. Some more severe patients will require oxygen at home. They may only need to use this during exertion, or they might require its use at all times.

In some cases, the patient may require short-term intubation or non-invasive ventilation (BiPap/CPAP).

Asthma

Asthma is another obstructive disease process and is defined by PubMed Health as: "a disorder that causes the airways of the lungs to swell and narrow, leading to wheezing, shortness of breath, chest tightness, and coughing."

Also, like COPD, asthma has been on the rise across the country. I don't know what it is about this disease, but in the years of doing this job, it amazes me how many people don't see how serious and deadly it is. Below are some facts from the Centers for Disease Control and Prevention:

- Number of non-institutionalized adults who currently have asthma: 18.7 million
- Number of children who currently have asthma: 7.0 million
- Number of visits (to physician offices, hospital outpatient and emergency departments) with asthma as primary diagnosis: 17.0 million
- Number of deaths per year: 3,388

Asthma is a disorder that when exposed to certain stimuli, a reaction occurs. This reaction can vary in severity, but at its basic, it causes the airways of the lungs to swell and constrict. The classic symptoms of an asthma attack are: wheezing, shortness of breath, chest tightness, and cough.

Numerous stimuli can lead to an asthma attack, and part of treating an asthma attack is to prevent it from occurring in the first place. Some testing can be done in an office, but the best way for a patient to understand what causes their attacks is by being a good historian. When symptoms start to present themselves, the patient should record when and where this occurred and list what type of environment they were in and possible irritants that may have been present. The more detailed the log, the better they will be able to identify and avoid situations which may flare an attack.

Pharmacological treatment of asthma may begin with anti-inflammatory agents or corticosteroids to help suppress the inflammatory process. Once the process has kicked in, it can be treated with bronchodilators and/or steroids. Supplemental oxygen may be needed and/or possibly intubation. Basically, you are to support whatever symptoms the patient presents themselves with. I will cover more about pharmacological agents later in this chapter.

Another invaluable tool for an asthmatic is a peak flow meter. The peak flow meter measures the speed at which someone can exhale and is measured in L/min. Each peak flow meter will come with a set of instructions. Within those instructions will be a guideline as to what the normal values should be for a person based on sex, age, and size. Don't get too hung up on these values as many patients' actual, best value might not fall within this range. It is also important for the patient to test themselves regularly at home during different times of the day until they can get a sense of what *their* normal value is.

Once a person's normal value is determined, the next step is setting "zones." Zones are percentages of the normal value achieved and are classified as the following:

- Green Zone   80-100% of normal   Safe
- Yellow Zone   60-80 % of normal   Acute Attack
- Red Zone   >60% of normal   Medical Alert

If the patient is in the red zone, they need to be seen in the emergency room right away. If the patient is in the yellow zone, they must begin whatever home regiment that is prescribed to them and should prepare to see a medical professional. An asthma attack can digress from yellow to red in a New York minute, and there is no time to waste seeking emergency help. We hear it all the time in the emergency room, "I didn't think it was that bad," or "I thought we had more time." Sometimes this is followed by a successful round of treatment for the patient, and other times it is after the patient has tragically died and the family laments about their decision to delay seeking treatment.

Obviously, it is very important for a patient to be able to learn the proper technique in performing a peak flow measurement. I have seen many patients in the emergency room over my career that have had peak flow meters and were not able to demonstrate how to use them correctly. Often times they have told me that the individual who gave this to them never instructed them. Patient education is paramount to the well-being of our asthmatic population.

The proper steps in performing a peak flow measurement from the asthmacenter.org are:

- Place the pointer at zero and hold the meter in a horizontal position in front of your mouth.
- Keep your fingers away from the pointer and vents of the meter.
- Empty your mouth of food or gum to avoid inhaling any foreign substance.
- Open your mouth and take in a slow, deep, maximum breath.
- Place your teeth on top of the mouthpiece and close your lips firmly around the mouthpiece so as not to permit any leaks.
- Forcefully blow out as fast as you can with an explosive breath in the shortest possible time.
- Observe your score and move the pointer back to zero and repeat the measurement in 30 seconds.
- Select the best reading of two or three efforts and record the results in your diary.
- If you have trouble using the peak flow meter because you are so short of breath or coughing a lot, it is time to increase your asthma medication and speak with your asthma specialist.

Treatment of asthma:

The treatment of asthma is very similar to that of COPD. If the patient can identify the stimuli that cause the reaction, great care should be used to avoid contact with the agent when possible.

Again, depending on the severity of the disease process, the asthma patient may be on any number of home medications. In some cases, the patient will only have to take the medication on an "as needed" basis. In other cases, they may need to take some medications routinely as a preventative measure. The following are a list of the common medications used in the treatment of asthma (covered more later):

<u>Bronchodilators</u>	<u>Corticosteroids</u>
Albuterol	Flovent
Atrovent	Solumedrol
Combivent	Prednisone
Spiriva	Advair
Theophylline	Budesonide
Xopenex	Flunisolide
Formoterol	Mometasone
Salmeterol	Beclomethasone

The similarities between COPD and asthma don't just end with medications. As with COPD, treatment of an asthmatic may require short-term oxygen, non-invasive ventilation, or intubation.

Sleep Apnea

Sleep apnea is a disorder where, during the time of sleep, the patient experiences either unusually shallow respirations and/or a complete interruption of breathing altogether. In many cases of sleep apnea, these events are not enough to warrant the need for intervention. Other cases are severe enough that it is vital for the patient to seek treatment. In these more severe cases, the interruption of breathing may actually cause the oxygen levels in the blood to drop to an unsafe level. Also, this continued interruption of sleep does not allow the patient to go into a deep, resting sleep (REM sleep). This leads to fatigue and drowsiness during the waking hours and can cause the same, if not worse, impairment during functions such as driving a vehicle or operating dangerous equipment.

Some facts about sleep apnea from yourlunghealth.org:

- Sleep apnea affects up to 18 million Americans.
- People with sleep apnea can stop breathing as many as 30 times or more each night.
- Officials estimate 10 million Americans have the condition but have not been diagnosed.
- Men, in general, suffer from sleep apnea more often than women.
- Studies have linked sleep apnea to high blood pressure, heart attack, and stroke.
- People with sleep apnea are three times more likely to be involved in motor vehicle accidents.
- People with sleep apnea sometimes fall asleep unexpectedly during the day, such as while talking on the phone or driving.
- Risk factors for sleep apnea include being overweight and having a large neck.
- Losing even 10% of body weight can help reduce the number of times a person with sleep apnea stops breathing during sleep.
- African-Americans, Pacific Islanders, and Mexican-Americans may be at increased risk for sleep apnea.
- Smoking and alcohol use increase the risk of sleep apnea.

There are two different types of sleep apnea: central and obstructive sleep apnea.

Central sleep apnea:

Central sleep apnea is when the patient stops breathing periodically during sleep because the brain temporarily stops sending signals to the muscles that control respiration. This can occur with patients who suffer from any variety of conditions, mostly neurological in nature.

Some of these conditions include: history of stroke, arthritis, degenerative bone and/or joint disease, spinal injuries, Parkinson's disease, and congestive heart failure.

Obstructive sleep apnea:

This is caused by a narrowing of a portion of the upper airway, most often due to obesity. Obesity causes an excess of soft tissue, which creates the obstruction. A few more rare causes of obstructive sleep apnea include tonsillar hypertrophy and certain skeletal deformities such as a small chin.

Occasionally, you might get an overlapping situation where the patient has a combination of both central and obstructive sleep apnea.

Proper diagnosis and treatment of sleep apnea requires a proper "sleep study" to be done, known as a polysomnogram, which should be performed at a qualified clinic. These clinics try to mimic a sleeping situation similar to that of your own home. The rooms used often resemble that of a fancy hotel room with cameras in place to monitor the patient's sleep. The patient is hooked up to a variety of monitors to measure chest movement, brain activity, oxygen levels, and other vital signs. A test like this simply can't be performed in a typical hospital setting. Improper lighting, noise levels, and uncomfortable beds do not replicate an ideal sleeping environment.

Even though it takes a formal sleep study to properly diagnose sleep apnea, a greater part of diagnosis does occur in an ordinary clinical/hospital setting. Some common signs of sleep apnea that are seen in the hospital are: decreased oxygen saturation when the patient is sleeping, snoring, visibly observing the patient stop breathing while asleep, and an obese patient with a large neck circumference.

The following are some of the questions you might want to ask the patient. If the patient has a spouse or significant other who sleeps in the same room with them, try to arrange the questionnaire when he or she is present. Sometimes the patient may not know the answers to some of the questions, or they may not give truthful answers:

- Do you snore?
- How loud do you snore?
- How often do you snore?
- Do you stop breathing when you sleep?
- Do you feel as if you didn't get adequate sleep when you wake up?
- Are you often times tired during the day?
- Do you doze off at work or while driving?
- Do you have high blood pressure?

Many times patients have one or more of these symptoms and don't relate it to the fact that they simply "snore" when sleeping.

Treatment of sleep apnea:

The most common treatment of sleep apnea is a home CPAP unit. There are also oral devices that can be placed in the mouth while sleeping. On some occasions, surgery might be an option. The normal surgical procedure is called uvulopalatopharyngo-plasty (say that five times fast!).

If a patient is admitted to the hospital and they are going to be there for one or more nights, it is important that we identify whether or not they have been previously diagnosed with sleep apnea. If so, you will want to find out if they sleep with a home CPAP machine. If they do, ask if they have it with them or if a family member or friend can get it for them. If they don't have it and can't get it, one must be provided for them by the facility. Often times these patients are admitted to general floor units and are not on continuous monitoring. Without the use of a CPAP machine, their oxygen levels could drop dangerously low, leading to outcomes that may be less than desirable.

4

Oxygen and Oxygen Delivery

T HE ADMINISTRATION OF OXYGEN IS A FAIRLY COMMON ORDER, and we see its use on many of our patients in the clinical setting. Understanding oxygen and its use, however, is not as simple as it may appear. Many times in my career I have seen oxygen systems set up incorrectly. I have seen oxygen used on patients who did not need it, and I have seen it not used when clearly indicated. Most of this, I believe, comes from a lack of understanding. My goal in this chapter is to get you to understand why we use oxygen and why we do not. How to set up the different oxygen devices and what can go wrong if they are set incorrectly is included in this chapter as well.

The indications for the use of oxygen are:

- Treatment of arterial hypoxemia
- Decreasing cardiopulmonary workload
- Decreasing work of breathing

Treatment of Arterial Hypoxemia

HYPOXEMIA: A condition where the oxygen level in the arterial blood is decreased below the normal predicted value of 80-100 mmHg.

One cause of hypoxemia might be a decrease in the oxygen content of the air we breathe. This does not happen often or naturally. It primarily happens in the case of a household or structural fire. Studies have shown that the FiO2 in an enclosed burning room can drop as low as 10 to 14% as the fire consumes the oxygen for fuel. Normal room air FiO2 is approximately 21%.

Common causes of arterial hypoxemia:

DEADSPACE VENTILATION: Occurs when the alveoli are filled with air/oxygen but are not getting perfused with blood. This can occur in cases such as hypovolemia, shock, and decreased blood pressure.

Hemoglobin deficiencies:

- Anemia
- Carboxyhemogolbinemia
- Methemogobinemia

PULMONARY SHUNT: Occurs when the alveoli are perfused with blood, but there is no air present for gas exchange to take place. It can happen when the alveoli are collapsed (atelectasis) or if they are filled with fluid such as in cases of pneumonia. There is also a certain amount of ventilation that occurs where the air does not make it to the alveolar level. This air does not make it past the upper airways and/or conductive airways, which makes it a normal anatomical pulmonary shunt. Pulmonary shunts can be exacerbated in cases of hypoventilation.

As mentioned previously, an oxygen saturation reading of 95 to 100% is a normal oximeter reading. Depending on your departmental guidelines and/or orders written by the physician, how low the oxygen saturation drops before administering supplemental oxygen can vary. Typically, it is 92% or lower. There are some conditions that our patient may have in which we would expect a less than normal reading, such as in COPD.

An arterial blood gas sample will provide us with the PaO_2, which, as mentioned earlier, has a normal value of 80 to 100 mm Hg.

The following is a case I was involved with: We had an elderly gentleman who spoke Spanish. He was a poor historian, so getting an accurate past medical history was not an option. His O_2 saturation was only 60 to 65%, yet he remained asymptomatic. We drew an arterial blood gas that showed a PAO_2 of 36. The pH and $PACO_2$ were fine. These oxygen numbers simply were not compatible with life, yet all other vitals were fine, and he was coherent and probably knew his surroundings better than us at that point. The conversation then consisted of, "How do we treat this?" We determined that those numbers were his baseline at home. It made no clinical sense, but we were going to treat the symptoms, not the numbers. This happened once before in my career where a man on room air had a baseline O_2 saturation of 75%, and he walked around and talked just as easy as any one of us. It is a valuable lesson. We treat symptoms, and we must understand our patients true baseline in order to treat him or her properly.

Decreasing Cardiopulmonary Workload

If the patient is tachycardic, supplemental oxygen is indicated. There are many reasons a patient may become tachycardic, one of which may be a lack of oxygen. If hypoxemia exists, the body tries to compensate for it. One of the compensatory mechanisms is for the heart rate to increase. The body realizes it has less oxygen in the blood stream than is required, so it tries to push the blood through the body faster in order to deliver the proper amount of oxygen. Thus, if we administer oxygen, it should correct the tachycardia. If there are other issues at hand creating the tachycardia, then oxygen is still indicated. If the blood is passing by the alveolar-capillary membrane faster than normal, it will have less time to get loaded up with oxygen. If there is more oxygen at the area of gas exchange, this may help keep the blood adequately oxygenated during this episode. The administration of oxygen may not help the tachycardia if the cause is not the lack of oxygen.

Decreasing Work of Breathing

If the patient has increased work of breathing, the administration of oxygen may be beneficial. An increased work of breathing could be demonstrated by: an increased respiratory rate, the use of accessory muscles, an increase in the depth of breathing, or a combination of all these factors. Often times, when the body is facing a hypoxic event, it will compensate by trying to pull more air in by breathing harder and faster. At some point, the patient may wear out and may not be able to keep up this work of breathing. Also, the harder the patient works, the more their O_2 consumption goes up. Our tissues need oxygen to live and function properly. If at any point the tissues are working harder, they will require (consume) more oxygen, thus O_2 consumption increases.

Risks of Oxygen Administration

Risks are involved with the administration of oxygen, so we want to be sure only to give oxygen when it is clearly indicated. Oxygen delivery does require a physician's order, so also make sure you have a clearly written order for what you are about to administer.

The following are some of the risks involved in the administration of oxygen:

ABSORPTION ATELECTASIS: Atelectasis is the partial and/or complete collapse of alveoli. The air we breathe contains about 21% oxygen and 78% nitrogen. Once the FiO_2 given to the patient exceeds 40%, the nitrogen starts to get flushed out of the lungs. Nitrogen does not absorb into the blood stream as well as oxygen. The nitrogen gas in the lungs could reduce the total volume of gas in the lungs and lead to atelectasis.

PRODUCTION OF FREE RADICALS: Without getting too technical, a free radical is basically a molecule that has a single, unpaired electron in an outer shell. Free radicals are very damaging to other structures of the body, including vital DNA and proteins. Free radicals basically destroy and kill healthy cells. Studies have shown that the delivery of too much oxygen releases more free radicals. How much is too much? Well, just like anything, there are a variety of opinions. What this means for us is that we must be vigilant about giving therapeutic oxygen when indicated and only as much as needed. We also must be aggressive in weaning our patients off of the oxygen as soon as the crises that warranted its use has ended.

KNOCKING OUT THE RESPIRATORY OR HYPOXIC DRIVE: All right, again, I'm going to try not to get too technical, but this one is a biggie. I touched on this topic earlier, now I'm going to devote a little more time to this as there is some controversy surrounding this risk factor. First, let's understand what knocking out the respiratory drive means. It basically means that if we give too much oxygen to a certain class of patients, they may stop breathing.

This is how that can happen: first of all, we have two main chemoreceptors that help regulate our breathing. Central chemoreceptors basically react to changes in the level of CO_2 in the system. An increase in CO_2 causes a reaction, which leads to an increase in depth and rate of breathing, thus lowering the CO_2 back to normal. Peripheral chemoreceptors are stimulated by PaO_2. A decreased PaO_2 sets off a reaction that leads to an increased depth of breathing, which corrects the hypoxemia.

The hypoxic drive theory states the following: patients that have the condition of Chronic Obstructive Pulmonary Disease (COPD) typically have a higher level of CO_2 due to their inability to breathe effectively. The central chemoreceptors gradually establish a higher baseline CO_2 as hypoventilation occurs, and CO_2 levels rise; the central chemoreceptors will fail to stimulate breathing. This leaves only the peripheral chemoreceptors to do the work. Since the peripheral chemoreceptors will trigger breathing based on a low level of PaO_2, if we give this type of patient too much supplemental oxygen and the PaO_2 doesn't drop, none of the chemoreceptors will send a signal telling the body to breathe. As I have said, this is controversy surrounding this topic. For a little bit more information on this controversy read Box 4-1.

FIRE HAZARD: Oxygen supports combustion, therefore making it easier to ignite a fire. It also fuels fire, causing the fire to burn stronger and longer. Despite the bombardment of education being done on this danger, there are still many needless fires and accidents involving an enriched oxygen environment.

Home oxygen users are warned not to smoke while on oxygen and yet: "In 2003-2006, hospital emergency rooms saw an estimated average of 1,190 thermal burns per year caused by ignitions associated with home medical oxygen." (nfpa.org)

Box 4-1

The Hypoxic Drive Theory: Fact Or Fiction?

Many articles have been written about this phenomenon, and the bottom line is that while hypoxic drive itself is true, the hypoxic drive theory is without a doubt in question. The proof behind the hypoxic drive theory came from studies showing ever-increasing levels of CO_2 when higher amounts of oxygen were delivered. The "debunkers" of this theory point out another effect called the Haldane Effect. The Haldane Effect states that when the hemoglobin of the blood has low amounts of oxygen, it has a greater ability to carry more CO_2. Thus, if the hemoglobin is over-saturated with oxygen, it carries less CO_2. This can lead to higher levels of CO_2 in the bloodstream and might be a bigger contributor to the increased CO_2 found in COPD patients receiving high amounts of supplemental oxygen.

So, what if we can't agree that this phenomenon is a myth and one wants to hold onto the idea that we can "knock out the hypoxic drive?" What then is the best way to treat a COPD patient who is in an exacerbation process? As I have quoted before: "Hypoxia kills; hypercapnia happens." So treat hypoxia.

Oxygen Delivery and Storage

There are a variety of ways in which oxygen is stored. You don't really need to know all the specifics of the storage options. The only one I want to tell you about is that of the oxygen tank.

We use oxygen tanks so that we can be more mobile with our patient. The tank or cylinder can be very dangerous if not handled correctly. Not only does oxygen pose a fire hazard, but when stored in a cylinder under high pressures, the tank can act as a missile if it is knocked over, which may cause the neck to break off. So, keeping these factors in mind, the following recommendations were made by the National Fire Protection Agency and the Compressed Gas Association.

- Store oxygen cylinders in a rack or chained against the wall.
- Store gas cylinders away from sources of heat.
- Keep full and empty tanks stored separately.
- Avoid dropping, dragging, or rolling cylinders in transport.

Many more regulations exist, but these are the highlights and the ones I see violated the most. If you see a cylinder standing unsecured in an upright position, secure it. If there is no way to secure the tank, then place it on its side. Placing an oxygen tank on its side is still not considered "safe", but it's far better than leaving it in an upright unsecured position.

Oxygen is delivered to the patient via a flow meter that is attached to the wall. Most flow meters can be adjusted from 0 to 15 L/min. From the flow meter there is usually a humidifier device or oxygen adapter (a.k.a. christmas tree adapter) connected. Always make sure these adapters are screwed on securely. A loose fitting adapter can create leaks, and your patient might not be getting the flow that is desired.

Medical gases are color-coded. The color associated with oxygen is green, so you will notice that all of the devices I just discussed are green in color: the knob on the flow meter, the christmas tree adapter, and the wall outlets. The other common gas seen in a patient room is that of compressed gas, or medical air.

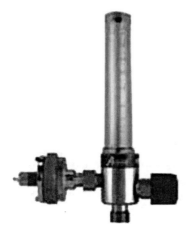

Oxygen Flow Meter

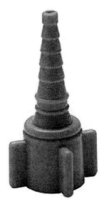

Christmas Tree

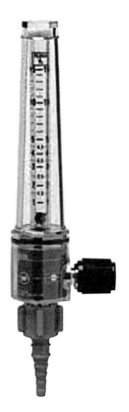

Flow Meter with
Christmas Tree

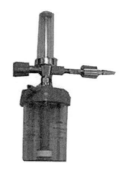

Flow Meter with
Humidification

This is yellow. Always be sure that when hooking up a device, you hook it up to a green flow meter and not a yellow one.

Oxygen delivery devices can be classified into two categories: low-flow or high-flow.

Low-Flow Oxygen Systems

These are systems that don't necessarily meet the inspiratory flow demands of a patient. They provide supplemental oxygen and are good devices for a patient who needs the oxygen for one of the reasons mentioned previously, but he or she is not extremely short of breath or working hard to breathe. These devices don't exceed 10 L/min of total flow, and the normal inspiratory flow is greater than 10 L/min. The following are the most commonly used low-flow oxygen systems:

NASAL CANNULA: Typically runs from 1 to 6 L/min, delivering 24 to 44% oxygen.

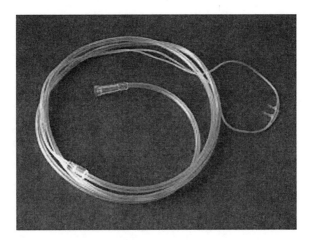

Nasal Cannula

The way to determine what approximate percentage of oxygen the patient is receiving is by using the following formula. Remembering that room air consists of roughly 21% oxygen, 1 L/min equals 24% oxygen. For every liter after 1, just add 4%.

1 L/min = 24%
2 L/min = 28%
3 L/min = 32%
4 L/min = 36%
5 L/min = 40%
6 L/min = 44%

I say that these are approximate percentages because they can vary depending on the patient's breathing pattern. The patient typically is breathing both through the mouth and nose, thus the patient is not only getting the oxygen via the nasal cannula, but is also entraining some room air with it. So if the patient is on 3 L/min (32%), but that is being mixed with room air (21%), the 32% will get diluted. The harder someone is breathing, the more room air will be entrained, and the less accurate the percentage delivered will be.

NASAL CATHETER: This is not used very often. Primarily, it's used during a procedure such as a bronchoscopy where using a nasal cannula would be difficult since the scope would be taking up 1 nare. It may also be used in someone needing long-term oxygen who might be experiencing skin breakdown from a nasal cannula, although I have rarely seen this used for such a purpose. Because it is inserted so far into the nares, it does create a comfort issue, which is the primary reason why it is not used more often. Just like the nasal cannula, it runs from 1 to 6 L/min, and the percentages of oxygen delivered are the same.

To insert, you first measure the catheter from nose to ear. It is then lubricated and inserted into a position just above the uvula.

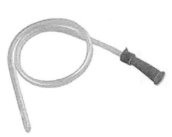 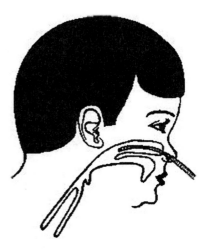

Nasal Catheter   Nasal Catheter Insertion

TRANSTRACHEAL CATHETER: The transtracheal catheter is a flexible tube, similar to a nasal catheter, which is inserted surgically through the neck, directly into the trachea. This is typically used for a patient using long term oxygen at home.

Some of the benefits of this system are as follows:

- More comfortable than a nasal cannula, less skin breakdown around the ears.
- Lower oxygen requirements. Since the oxygen is being delivered right where it is needed, O_2 requirements can be up to 50 to 60% lower (www.tto.com).
- Improved self-image. Sometimes it is uncomfortable for a patient to go in public wearing a nasal cannula.

Disadvantages of transtracheal oxygen:

- It does have to be inserted surgically.
- Greater risk of infection.
- Requires greater care in cleaning and maintaining.

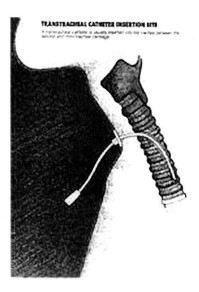

Transtracheal Catheter

RESERVOIR CANNULAS: As its name suggests, this is a nasal cannula with a built-in reservoir. Whereas we normally think of a reservoir as a storage facility for water, in this case it is a storage facility for oxygen. What this allows for is the ability to give the patient a larger percentage of oxygen via a nasal cannula. When the patient breathes in, they are not only getting oxygen from the wall or tank source, but they are also drawing in more oxygen via the reservoir.

Some examples of the nasal reservoir:

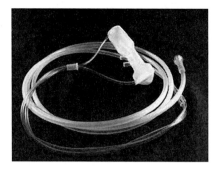

Nasal Cannula Reservoir

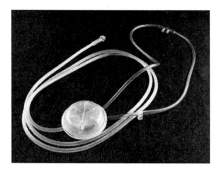

Nasal Cannula
Pendant Reservoir

SIMPLE MASK: Runs at 5 to 12 L/min and delivers 35 to 55% oxygen. It is important not to run this mask at less than 5 L/min. As a patient exhales, they are exhaling CO_2. The CO_2 will be exhaled into the mask. The mask needs at least 5 L/min of oxygen flowing through it to flush out the CO_2. If the flow is not enough, the patient will rebreathe the CO_2, leading to hypercapnea.

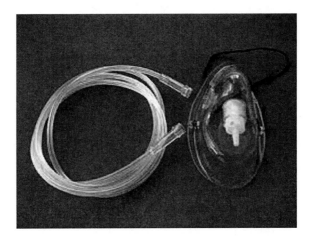

Simple Oxygen Mask

PARTIAL REBREATHING MASK: Runs at 8 to 15 L/min and delivers 35 to 60% oxygen. The partial rebreathing mask has a bag attached, which is a reservoir similar to the reservoir discussed previously with the nasal cannula. This reservoir allows the patient to draw oxygen from it when the flow from the wall or oxygen tank is not enough to meet the patient's inspiratory requirements. It is important that when the patient breathes in, the bag does not completely collapse. This means the flow from the flow meter is not high enough and needs to be turned up. Ideally, the bag should remain 1/3 to ½ full.

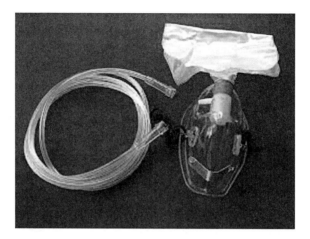

Partial Rebreathing Mask

NONREBREATHING MASK: This mask is very similar to the partial rebreathing mask but will deliver a greater percentage of oxygen. It runs from 8 to 15 L/min and delivers 60 to 90% oxygen. The same rules apply regarding the reservoir bag not collapsing upon inspiration.

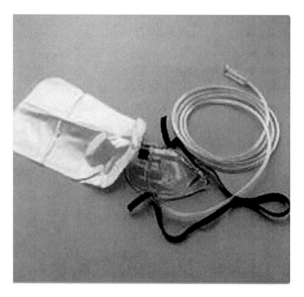

Non Rebreathing Mask

High-Flow Oxygen Systems

These basically provide a high enough oxygen concentration at a flow that either equals or exceeds the patient's peak inspiratory flow. The peak inspiratory flow varies from patient to patient. It will also vary with the same patient, depending on their changing respiratory demands. If a condition occurs that causes the work of breathing to rise significantly, then the peak inspiratory flow the patient needs will rise as well. If the patient is on one of the previously mentioned low-flow sources and it is not correcting the work of breathing, then consider a high-flow source.

VENTURI MASK: This mask delivers 24 to 50% oxygen to the patient. It is also known as an air-entrainment system. There are currently two common styles of venturi masks on the market (see the image below). The first one has a dial attached to the mask. Along one side of the dial are percentages of oxygen coupled with an associated liter flow. The other side of the dial has a little window. The window allows air from the atmosphere to enter, or be entrained, into the flow of oxygen. The mixture of oxygen from the oxygen source and the amount of air entrained will determine the percentage of oxygen the patient is receiving. As you turn the dial to a higher percentage of oxygen, the window will get smaller, thus allowing less atmospheric oxygen (21%) to mix with the flow of oxygen from the wall or tank, which increases the percent of oxygen delivered to the patient. The other design uses various colored adaptors that can be connected to the mask. Each colored adaptor is marked with how much oxygen will be delivered and what the liter flow should be coming from the oxygen source.

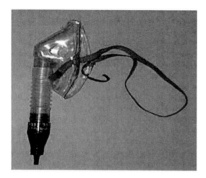

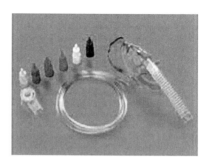

Venturi Mask System   Venturi Mask System

AEROSOL MASK: It's not so much the mask, but the system it is connected to. The mask is connected to a high-flow air, humidified, air entrainment device. There are too many of these devices to list or show images of, but the picture provided shows a system with most of the common features.

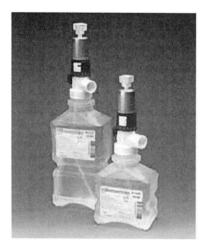

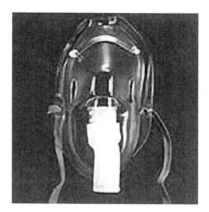

High-Flow Aerosol Set Up   Aerosol Mask

The top of the system attaches to the oxygen flow meter. There is a blue dial that, like the venturi mask, can be turned to adjust the percentage of oxygen. The dial has the percentages marked on it and the same "window" that the venturi mask had.

The humidification bottle attached to the system allows you to deliver humidified air to the patient. The humidification is an important aspect. Our lungs need humidification. With such a high flow of dry air being delivered to the patient, the nasal mucosa can dry out, and the secretions in the lungs could become thicker and harder to expectorate.

FACE TENT: The face tent is used the same way as the aerosol mask. It attaches to the same system featured above. As you can tell from the picture, the face tent does not cover the face but instead forms a large "tent" formation resting on the chin. You would use this type of mask on a patient who can't tolerate a face mask. If a person is claustrophobic, they may feel like they are actually suffocating with an aerosol mask. Another reason to use the fact tent would be in the case of facial trauma, such as: fractures, lacerations, or burns. The mask could be painful and may exacerbate the injuries.

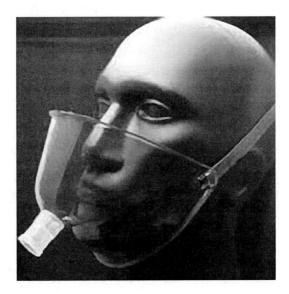

Face Tent

Trach mask: Works just like an aerosol mask or face tent. Again, it attaches to the same system as above. This mask is used for a patient with an artificial airway called a tracheostomy. It is essential that the trach mask is always attached to a proper humidification system. Remember that one of the functions of the upper airways is to humidify. The upper airway exchange system typically adds about one liter of humidification to the lower airways a day. When the upper airway is bypassed, either by an endotracheal tube or a tracheostomy, the body loses that function. If proper humidification is not supplied, the lower airways get dry.

The most common complication in a situation such as this is mucus plugging. Mucus plugging can become severe enough to occlude the entire airway and can result in death. I have seen more mucus plugging on trach patients than I care to recollect, and often times it is a direct result of improper humidification. Even if the patient does not require oxygen, they should still be wearing a trach mask with the system connected to medical air. While connected to medical air, it does not matter what the percentage of oxygen says on the dial, the patient is always receiving 21%, or room air.

The big question is usually, "What delivery device should I choose?" Remember the purpose for providing the oxygen to

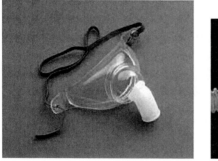

Trach Mask

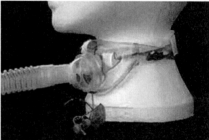

Trach Mask

begin with. Your goal is to choose the system that provides the appropriate amount of oxygen to correct the problem. Second, you want to use the device that provides sufficient flow to meet the patient's inspiratory (work of breathing) demands and one that feels comfortable for the patient. This all requires assessment and reassessment. You may have to use various adjuncts throughout the day to meet the changing requirements of your patient. Of course, the last factor in determining what system to use would be what is available at the facility you work at. Not every facility has every adjunct, so you need to be familiar with what is provided where you work and how to use it.

Troubleshooting

If your patient is receiving supplemental oxygen and you notice his or her oxygen saturation is below normal, yet they appear fine/asymptomatic, double check your equipment. Make sure that device is hooked up to an oxygen flow meter. Sometimes it becomes disconnected or is accidentally connected to a yellow flow meter, which is simply compressed air and not oxygen. Follow the line from the wall to the patient. Make sure it is not kinked off or disconnected somewhere. Check to be sure it is on the patient correctly. Once all is in working order and the saturation is still an issue, then you can consider escalating the amount of oxygen the patient should receive.

There are many types of humidification bottles that can be used with the oxygen devices. Some of the bottles can only handle a low flow of oxygen and can't support the higher flows required for one of the oxygen mask systems mentioned previously. If you are unsure whether the humidification device is compatible with the oxygen device, check with someone from respiratory.

5

Respiratory Therapy Treatments

THERE ARE A VARIETY OF TREATMENTS TO COMBAT RESPIRATORY complications at our disposal. I want to cover the most common treatments used today. In an era of cost-containment, there has been more cross training, and in some facilities nurses are asked to perform some of the treatments I will be discussing. To this end, I will be sure to point out proper techniques and common errors I see when these treatments are administered. It is vital that we perform and educate the patient to perform the techniques properly. Improper techniques can lead to subpar results and increased patient stay and cost.

You must also understand the indications and contraindications for the treatment. As I mentioned before, cross training is more common in the hospital setting than it once was. Even if you don't perform the task, you might be the one who suggests to the physician a treatment you think will be beneficial to the patient. You might be a physician, physician's assistant, or nurse practitioner who has the ability to order the treatment, in which case a better understanding of the modality is paramount to patient outcome.

50

Metered Dose Inhaler (MDI)

This is the most commonly prescribed method of aerosolized drug therapy. Its biggest advantage to other modalities is that it is quick, easy to perform, and the inhaler is small enough to carry with you. It does, however, require a bit of coordination to perform correctly. The side effects of this and other delivery methods of aerosolized medications are primarily limited to the medication itself and not the method used to deliver it.

As I review the technique of performing the MDI, I think it is important to point out that as many as two-thirds of patients and/or health professionals perform this task improperly (Egan's Fundamentals of Respiratory Care, pg. 808). For this reason, as I mention the steps, I will include why each step is important. I use the same explanation when instructing my patients. I find that if they understand why the steps are important, they are more apt to follow them:

1. Sit or stand up straight, slightly lift the chin to open the airways. The medication must make its way from the device, through the mouth, past the upper airways, and all the way down to the lower airways. Proper posture will allow for the patient to take a deeper breath in, and the slightly raised chin will provide a more direct path.

2. Before using an MDI for the first time, or if it has not been used for several days, prime it by pointing the MDI into the air, away from people, and actuating it. Often times the first "puff" of medication does not actually carry a full dose. By priming the inhaler, the patient will receive a full dose on the next "puff."

3. Remove the cap from the mouthpiece and attach it to a spacer device (covered later in the chapter), if provided. I guess it goes without saying that if the mouthpiece is still intact, the patient won't get the medication no matter

how many times they actuate the inhaler. This may sound funny, but I have seen it happen.

It is important to note that there are two techniques taught: the open mouth and closed mouth technique. There is literature to support both methods, so I recommend doing whatever the patient is able to perform best.

4. Take a few deep breaths and then breathe out gently.
5. **Open mouth technique:** Open your mouth wide while keeping your tongue down. Hold the MDI about 4 cm away from your mouth.
6. **Closed mouth technique:** Place the mouthpiece in your mouth and put your teeth around it. Seal your lips around the mouthpiece, holding it between your lips.
7. Start to breathe in slowly and deeply. As you start to breathe in, press down on the canister to release the medication. This ensures that when the inhaler is activated, the medication will enter the inspiratory flow already in progress, thus maximizing the amount of medication received. If it is activated prior to the breath being initiated, the medication will enter static airflow and will be lost.
8. Continue to breathe in as deeply as you can. The deeper you breathe in, the deeper the medication will be distributed, thus maximizing its deposition.
9. Hold your breath for 10 seconds, if possible. Often times I have seen a patient inhale the medication and breathe out right away. Remember that this medication is aerosolized. By holding your breath, it will allow the medication time to settle into the airways. Exhaling too quickly will simple be blowing the medication right back out from where it came.

10. If a second puff is needed, wait for at least one minute before taking the next puff. This is more important with a fast-acting bronchodilator, such as albuterol, than with any other medication. However, it is an important rule to follow at all times. By waiting one minute, it gives the patient time to "reset" their breathing, so they can follow all of the above techniques optimally. As for the case with albuterol, it is a fast-acting medication. By simply waiting one minute, this medication will already start opening up some of the airways. This means the second dose should be able to be deposited deeper into the airways, creating a better result. If the two puffs are taken back to back, the medication simply goes the same depth and is not as effective.

A **spacer** is a large, cylindrical device that has two openings. One opening connects to the MDI, while the other opening is shaped into a mouthpiece. The spacer can simplify the use of the MDI as it is easier to hold onto and does not require as much coordination. It also provides a more direct path for the medication, so not as much of it will be lost into the oropharynx (mouth).

A study documented in the CHEST Journal showed the following results when comparing patients using an MDI with and without a chamber:

"There was a statistically greater improvement in peak flow rates in the MDI/spacer group (126.8 vs. 111.9 L/min, respectively; $p = 0.002$). The MDI/spacer group also spent significantly less time in the ED (163.6 and 175 min, respectively; $p = 0.007$), had a lower total albuterol dose (1,125 μg and 6,700 μg, respectively; $p < 0.001$), and showed a greater improvement in arterial oxygen saturation ($p = 0.043$). Relapse rates at 14 and 21 days were significantly lower ($p < 0.01$ and $p < 0.05$, respectively) among patients treated with the MDI/spacer and were associated with asthma education and the provision of a peak flow meter, a spacer, and an inhaled corticosteroid for patients' home use."

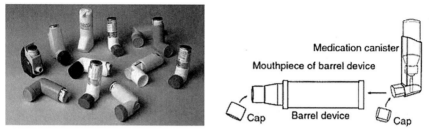

MDI   MDI with Spacer

(A Comparison of Albuterol Administered by Metered-Dose Inhaler and Spacer With Albuterol by Nebulizer in Adults Presenting to an Urban Emergency Department with Acute Asthma; Kenneth B. Newman, MD, FCCP; Scott Miline, MD; Cathy Hamilton, MPH; Kent Hall, MD.)

Dry Powdered Inhalers

This type of inhaler is very similar to that of an MDI. In fact, the technique for delivery is relatively the same. The biggest difference is the form in which the medication is produced. As its name suggests, this type of medication comes in the form of a dry powder. This makes the inhaler "gravity dependent." In a typical, liquid-style MDI, no matter how you hold the inhaler, the medication will not "leak out." It is not dispersed until you push down on the canister. In the dry powdered form, you must "activate" the medication by either pushing down on a canister or sliding a mechanism. In both cases, the capsule within the inhaler is punctured, allowing for the release of the powder. The powder will just sit in there until it is drawn into the airways by the patient inhaling on the device or if the device is tipped in a manner where the mouthpiece is facing the floor. Gravity will ensue, and the medication will fall out.

The steps for a dry powdered inhaler are as follows:

1. Load the dose.
2. Exhale slowly.

3. Seal your lips around the mouthpiece.

4. Inhale forcefully and as deep as possible.

5. Hold your breath for up to 10 seconds, if possible.

6. Repeat the process if more than one puff is directed.

A spacer is not used when administering a dry powdered inhaler. Also remember, if you are giving a steroid via an inhaler,

---

Myths and Misconceptions

The most common medication delivered via MDI or Nebulizer is albuterol. Albuterol is a bronchodilator. It opens constricted airways, and that is basically all it does. Through my years of experience, I have seen "breathing treatments" with albuterol ordered for many of the wrong reasons, such as:

The patient's O2 sat is low
The patient is short of breath
To "thin out secretions"
The patient has a cough
The patient smokes
The patient has a pleural effusion
The patient is unresponsive
The patient has broken ribs
The patient has a history of COPD and/or asthma

I'm sure if I asked my fellow therapists, I'd be able to double the list. The point is this: unless any of the above-mentioned problems are caused by bronchoconstriction, then giving a breathing treatment with albuterol will not help. It will not drain a pleural effusion, wake someone up, and is not necessary for a patient with a history of COPD and /or asthma unless they are symptomatic. Many studies have been published regarding the over ordering of this medication with results anywhere from 12 to 50%

have the patient rinse their mouth out after use. If remnants of the steroid remain in the mouth, it could lead to thrush.

Hand Held Nebulizer

This is "the breathing treatment." First, you place a liquid medication into a holding device, which is then connected to a gas source such as oxygen or compressed air. The flow is then turned on, and as the flow of air passes over the liquid, it draws the liquid into the flow of air, creating a "mist." This mist is directed toward a mouthpiece for the patient to inhale. The mouthpiece can be substituted with an aerosol mask for those patients who cannot hold onto the mouthpiece or a trach mask for those with an artificial airway.

Let me describe this to you in the way I typically describe it to a patient:

"I am going to give you a breathing treatment. After I assemble the equipment and hand it to you, you will see that it looks like a funny pipe that you smoke. You simply place the mouthpiece of the pipe into your mouth and breathe nice and easy through your mouth. I don't want you working real hard on this because the treatment lasts 5 to 10 minutes, and I don't want you to wear yourself out. I want you to take in a bigger breath and hold it for a few seconds about every fourth breath or so. This will help you get more medication without wearing yourself out. The mist you see coming from this pipe is the medication (I will go on to explain more about the particular medication I am giving at this point, along with common side effects). If at any point you don't feel well, just let me know, and we can stop the treatment."

Most of the medications that are delivered via MDI can also be delivered via a hand held nebulizer. There are many reports, studies, and research done as to what is more effective, the MDI or the nebulizer. There are enough studies to basically state that it is still up to debate. Some say one delivers more medication than the other. Some state that one or the other is more cost effective.

I believe that the best way to determine how to deliver the medication is to ask and/or evaluate the patient. If they have a home regiment that involves nothing but the use of an MDI, then that is the method we should stick with so long as they are able to use the proper technique. If, while observing, the patient appears to be able to do one technique better than another, then that is the way we should administer it. Despite all of the studies done, the best answer is always the same to me: it's patient dependent.

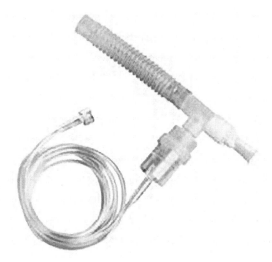

Hand Held Nebulizer

Incentive Spirometry (I.S.)

Incentive spirometry is a therapy that is used for the purpose of lung expansion. The primary reason a patient may need lung expansion therapy is to prevent and/or treat atelectasis.

ATELECTASIS: is the collapse of part of the lung, or in some rare cases, the entire lung. A few of the more common reasons for atelectasis to occur are:

- Mucus plugging that can prevent air from getting to parts of the lung distal to the plug.

- A consistent, shallow respiratory pattern from the patient. This may be caused by anesthetics or as a protective mechanism due to pain.
- Prolonged bed rest.
- May result from the use of anesthesia gases.

INCENTIVE SPIROMETRY: is designed to mimic the natural sighs a person takes during their regular day. During the therapy, the patient is instructed to take slow, deep breaths while observing the device that has different monitoring cues, which inform the patient of how they are performing.

Indications include: presence of atelectasis (usually confirmed via chest x-ray) or conditions that may lead to atelectasis.

Contraindications primarily only include patients who simply can't or won't perform the therapy. Sometimes we may not

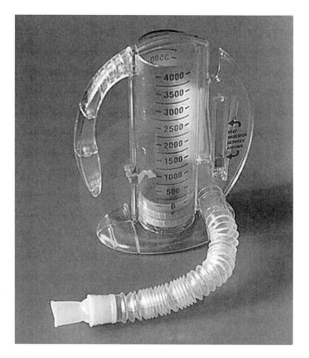

Incentive Spirometer

administer this therapy if the patient is on high-flow oxygen and disrupting this flow would cause a rapid drop in the patient's O_2 saturation.

Most incentive spirometers have two indicators on them. One indicator shows the amount of air being breathed into the lungs. The second indicator represents the speed being breathed in. There are usually two arrows where the speed is indicated, and the goal is to breathe in at a speed where the flow indicator hovers between the two arrows. The proper technique for incentive spirometer:

1. Sit or lie in a comfortable position with the best posture that can be tolerated.
2. Slide the volume indicator to the desired level. For example, start at 1500 ml and slowly increase as your treatment improves.
3. Hold the incentive spirometer in the upright position.
4. Place the mouthpiece into your mouth and close your mouth tightly around it (a nose clip can be used to create a better result).
5. Take a slow deep breath in.
6. Hold your breath for 3 seconds, if possible.
7. Allow the volume indictor to drop back to the bottom before taking the next breath.
8. Perform 1 set of 10 repetitions every hour followed by a good cough.

Intermittent Positive Pressure Breathing (IPPB)

Like incentive spirometry, IPPB is also indicated for the use of lung expansion. An IPPB machine is a machine that can deliver a positive pressure breath to a spontaneously breathing patient. A circuit is connected to the machine. On one end of the circuit is a mouthpiece. The patient places the mouthpiece in their mouth and closes his or her mouth tightly around the mouthpiece. As the patient breathes in, the machine senses the inspiratory flow and "cycles" a breath, pushing air into the lungs with the intention of expanding the collapsed airways. As the patient exhales against the machine, the machine will stop the flow of the air, allowing the patient to effectively exhale.

A nebulizer cup is also built into the circuit. This nebulizer can be filled with normal saline, or a liquid medication may be placed in it so that the patient is not only getting the benefit of the positive pressure breath, but is also getting the benefit of the nebulized medication being delivered deep into the airways.

The IPPB is indicated for patients who can't perform the incentive spirometer effectively. It is also good for patients with a weak, ineffective cough who are having issues with secretion management. The circuit can be adapted to deliver the treatment via a trach.

Contraindications include:

- Untreated tension pneumothorax
- Intracranial pressure (ICP) > 15 mm Hg
- Hemodynamic instability
- Recent facial, oral, or face surgery
- Tracheoesophageal fistula
- Recent esophageal surgery
- Active hemoptysis
- Nausea
- Active untreated tuberculosis
- Radiographic evidence of bleb
- Singultus (hiccups)

Hazards/Complications include:

- Barotrauma/pneumothorax
- Hemoptysis

- Gastric distention
- Secretion impaction (inadequate humidity)
- Impedance of venous return
- Air trapping, auto-PEEP, over distended alveoli

(AARC Clinical Practice Guidelines, AARC.org)

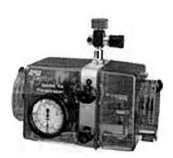

IPPB

Postural Drainage and Percussion

Postural drainage is usually talked about separately from percussion, but for the purposes of this text, I'm going to combine the two.

POSTURAL DRAINAGE THERAPY: involves placing the patient in different positions, thus altering the position of the lungs and allowing gravity to assist in the removal of secretions.

PERCUSSION: is typically performed along with postural drainage to maximize the benefits. Percussion involves rhythmically striking the chest wall in a fashion to "knock loose" thick secretions from the chest wall, therefore making it easier for them to be expectorated.

Percussion can either be done manually with a cupped hand, or with specifically designed machines. Usually, respiratory therapists and/or physical therapists conduct this therapy. I have never heard of any other group of health care professionals performing this. That is not to say that there aren't, but I believe it is such a small percentage that I will not go into great detail about how to conduct such a therapy.

Postural drainage alone involves twelve different positions the patient can be placed in and is decided based on where in the pulmonary structure the secretion problem is occurring. The process of percussion takes time to perfect, and since it is a process of actually "striking," the patient harm can be caused if not done correctly.

Postural drainage and percussion indications:

- Poor oxygenation associated with position
- Potential for or presence of atelectasis related to secretions
- Evidence or suggestion of difficulty with secretion clearance
- Evidence or suggestion of retained secretions in the presence of an artificial airway
- Diagnosis of diseases such as: cystic fibrosis, bronchiectasis, or cavitating lung disease

Postural drainage and percussion contraindications:

- Unstable head and/or neck injury
- Active hemorrhage with hemodynamic instability
- Intracranial pressure (ICP > 20 mm Hg)
- Recent spinal surgery or acute spinal injury
- Active hemoptysis
- Empyema
- Pulmonary edema associated with congestive heart failure
- Pulmonary embolism

- Rib fracture, with or without flail chest
- Surgical wound or healing tissue
- Large pleural effusions
- Subcutaneous emphysema
- Recent epidural spinal infusion or spinal anesthesia
- Recently placed transvenous pacemaker or subcutaneous pacemaker
- Pulmonary contusion
- Recent skin grafts, or flaps, on the thorax
- Burns, open wounds, and skin infections of the thorax
- Suspected pulmonary tuberculosis
- Bronchospasm
- Complaints of chest wall pain

Postural drainage and percussion complications:

- Hypoxemia
- Increased ICP
- Acute hypotension during procedure
- Pulmonary hemorrhage
- Pain or injury to muscles, ribs, or spine
- Vomiting and aspiration
- Bronchospasm
- Arrhythmias

(AARC Clinical Practice Guidelines, AARC.org)

Respiratory Pharmacology

The purpose of this section is to give you a brief overview or summary of the common respiratory medications used today. I'm not going to get into the dosing and all of the side effects. The goal at the end of this section is to provide you with the basic information, so the medications and their usage will not seem quite so foreign to you.

ADRENERGIC BRONCHODILATORS: are the most commonly used respiratory medications and are indicated for the presence of reversible airflow obstruction, such as in the cases of: asthma, bronchitis, emphysema, and COPD. This group of drugs is further broken down into **short-acting agents** and **long-acting agents.**

SHORT-ACTING AGENTS: are also known as "rescue drugs." They typically provide immediate relief of acute reversible airflow obstruction in asthma and COPD. The two primary drugs in this group would be albuterol and levalbuterol.

Drug	Brand Name
Albuterol	Proventil, Ventolin, AccuNeb
Levalbuterol	Xopenex

So, what this means is, if you have a patient who is having an asthma attack or is suffering from an exacerbation of their COPD, these are the drugs you want to use first to try and achieve immediate relief of the symptoms presented.

RACEMIC EPINEPHRINE: is another medication that falls under the classification of a short-acting agent. I mention it separately because its indications for use are different than albuterol and levalbuterol.

Racemic epinephrine is used for its ability to reduce upper airway swelling. It can sometimes be difficult to assess, but when a patient is wheezing, it is not always coming from the lower airways. If there is a component of upper airway inflammation, it can create a similar wheezing sound. This sound can resonate throughout the lower airways, thus "tricking" us into believing that this is where the origin of the problem is located. Albuterol and levalbuterol will not fix the problem if it originates in the upper airways. This upper airway "wheezing" may be different in tone and can be classified as stridor, mentioned earlier.

Drug	Brand Name
Racemic Epinephrine	MicroNefrin, Nephron

Long-acting agents are also bronchodilators, but they take a longer time to "kick in." They should not be used as "rescue" drugs; rather, they are used for maintenance. They help to prevent or control the bronchospasms. Some of the common drugs that fall under this classification are: salmeterol, formoterol, and arformoterol.

Drug	Brand Name
Salmeterol	Serevent
Formoterol	Foradil
Arformoterol	Brovana

ANTICHOLINERGIC BRONCHODILATORS: work by blocking cholinergic-induced bronchoconstriction. Again, these are not meant as "rescue" drugs but are used to help prevent the bronchoconstriction from occurring. The drugs used in this category are Ipratopium Bromide and Tiotropium Bromide.

Drug	Brand Name
Ipratopium Bromide	Atrovent
Tiotropium Bromide	Spiriva

Mucolytics

A mucolytic is designed to thin out secretions. There are currently two types of mucolytics on the market today, and both are designed to counter a different kind of mucus.

ACETYLCYSTEINE: is indicated to reduce the buildup of secretions in the airways. This medication is part of the sulpha group, so it is not indicated for a patient who is allergic to sulpha medications. Also, it can cause bronchospasms, so it should be given with albuterol or levalbuterol to minimize the risk.

DORNASE ALFA: works by breaking down the DNA material from neutrophils found in purulent secretions. Not all secretions have this characteristic. This particular type of secretion is most prevalent in patients with a condition called cystic fibrosis.

Drug	Brand Name
Acetylcysteine	Mucomyst
Dornase Alfa	Pulmozyme

INHALED CORTICOSTEROIDS: are anti-inflammatory agents and are meant as a maintenance therapy for patients with asthma and severe COPD. Maintenance means that the patient takes this medication on a scheduled basis. It usually takes time for the medication to "build up" in the system so that it is at a therapeutic level. I have seen these drugs ordered as "PRN for shortness of breath" on occasion. This is an incorrect order and not the way this particular class of medications was meant to be used. There is quite a long list of drugs that fall under this class, and I have them listed below:

Drug	Brand Name
Beclomethasone	QVAR
Triamcinolone Acetonide	Azmacort
Flunisolide	AeroBid
Fluticasone Propionate	Flovent
Budesonide	Pulmicort
Fluticasone Propionate/Salmeterol	Advair
Budesonide/Formoterol Fumarate	Symbicort

6

Respiratory Failure and Airway Management

RESPIRATORY FAILURE: is any condition that inhibits the normal delivery of oxygen to the tissues or inhibits the removal of carbon dioxide from the tissues.

There are two types of respiratory failure:

HYPOXEMIC RESPIRATORY FAILURE: occurs when the primary problem is the delivery of oxygen to the tissues.

HYPERCAPNIC RESPIRATORY FAILURE: occurs when the primary problem is the elimination of carbon dioxide, or a ventilation issue.

It is common to see patients experiencing both types of respiratory failure simultaneously.

Clinically, there has been an established guideline based on the results of an arterial blood gas to determine if a patient is within the limits of respiratory failure. The commonly recognized value would be a $PaCO_2 > 55$ with a corresponding pH of < 7.35. Hypoxic respiratory failure is defined as a PaO_2/FIO_2 < 200 also known as the P to F ratio.

Clinical numbers and guidelines are fine, but it doesn't take away the most important component of determining respiratory failure, and that is good clinical observation. I mentioned it before, and I'll say it again, nothing matches our good assessment skills.

There are some common sense things that we need to observe: work of breathing, respiratory rate, heart rate, and blood pressure. All of these vital signs can give us an indication as to whether or not our patient might be heading toward respiratory failure. And again, we need to know our patient's baseline status. If we don't know what is normal for our particular patient, then we don't know what is abnormal.

Many COPD patients have a chronically high $PaCO_2$, so a $PaCO_2$ level above 55 may not be out of the ordinary for this patient. I once worked with an attending physician who used to always ask, "Is your patient getting better? Are they getting worse? Or are they the same?" Without the answer to these questions, we can't determine if the patient is heading toward respiratory failure. It is not enough to know where the patient is right now; we have to know where they came from. This is also known as trending.

Typically, as a patient's pulmonary status gets worse, you will see the respiratory rate increase. You may note an increase in the work of breathing. If the patient is asthmatic, you may hear wheezes upon auscultation of the chest. As the problem gets worse and the patient starts to wear out, the respiratory rate will start to get lower, and the work of breathing will not appear to be as labored since the patient has no effort to give anymore. And where we once heard wheezing, we may hear little to no air exchange. Diminished breath sounds in an asthmatic patient are not always good. Sometimes it means that the airways are so constricted that you can't even hear the wheezing anymore.

Again, the above scenario shows what you would recognize if you have been "trending" the patient's signs and symptoms. If you were not and just looked at the end result (prior to the code), you might miss valuable information.

Once we have determined that a patient's pulmonary condition is on the decline, we must decide on an appropriate course of action. The ultimate goal is to treat the condition in the least invasive fashion as possible. Below is a list of options from least to most invasive, all of which we can choose for our patient to try to reverse the condition:

- Low-flow oxygen
- High-flow oxygen
- Use of an inhaler (provided the patient can still do a proper technique)
- Nebulizer breathing treatment (with presence of bronchoconstriction)
- IPPB
- Oral suctioning to clear out secretions
- Nasotracheal suctioning
- Non-invasive ventilation
- Intubation followed by mechanical ventilation

Keep in mind that this list consists of the respiratory modalities that can be used. Also keep in mind that in this list are the most commonly used adjuncts. There are a variety of equipment options available, but not every facility has access to them. It would take an entire book to cover every piece of equipment that exists.

I've already covered the first five options on the above list. The remaining choices all fall under the classification of airway management.

Airway Management

AIRWAY MANAGEMENT: is a vital role for everyone in the medical field. If it is neglected, what could have been an easy fix for the patient may soon become a life-threatening event. Knowing how to properly suction secretions out of a patient who has an ineffective cough is essential in the beginning discussions of airway management. Often times a patient is intubated too quickly without even giving non-invasive ventilation a chance.

With that being said, before we talk about non-invasive versus invasive ventilation, I need to talk to you about things you can do to attempt to avoid that scenario altogether.

Suctioning

SUCTIONING: involves using a device which produces a negative pressure, attaching a suction hose and an adaptor that will be introduced to the patient's airway. The goal is to remove anything that could be causing an airway obstruction.

Remember all those wonderful days spent at the dentist's office? Sometimes they would attach that "sucking" device to your mouth, so you wouldn't have to rinse and drool all over yourself. Well, that is what we are talking about. It is our job to ensure that the patient's airway remains clear of debris and is patent.

Suctioning can be done in just the mouth, or deeper suctioning can be performed by going through the nose and traveling past the trachea.

ORAL SUCTIONING: is usually performed with a rigid device commonly known as the Yankauer. You must be careful not to gag the patient or to apply the suction for too long as it could create a sore.

NASOTRACHEAL SUCTIONING: is a little more invasive. This procedure involves passing a suction catheter through the nose and advancing it into the lower airways. Because this is an invasive procedure, we must be sure to assess the need to perform it.

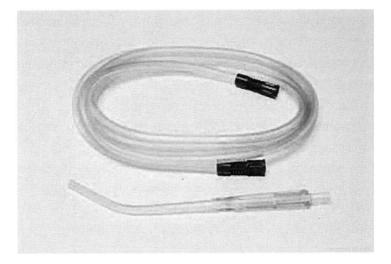

Yankauer

Indications that a patient needs nasotracheal suctioning would include those that have evidence of secretions in the lower airways, which the patient cannot effectively expectorate on their own. Now this alone is not a good reason to perform nasotracheal suctioning. If the patient is wide awake and the chest congestion does not appear to be creating a problem (in other words, the patient is asymptomatic), I'd be hesitant to perform this procedure. If however, the patient is in need of supplemental oxygen and their work of breathing has increased, I would then consider this to help improve their situation. Remember, this is invasive and uncomfortable for the patient; we don't just want to do this unless there are good indications.

You don't want to perform this procedure on someone who has facial fractures or recent surgery involving the face and/or nose. If the patient has occluded nasal passageways or epistaxis (nosebleed), you want to avoid giving nasotracheal suctioning.

In many facilities, it is required for a patient to be on a monitor when performing this task. Many complications can occur when performing nasotracheal suctioning, so you need to be prepared. Remember, when you suction out secretions from a patient's lungs, you are also sucking out air or oxygen. For this reason, it is good practice to pre-oxygenate the patient, especially if they have been having periods of hypoxic events. Also, this procedure can stimulate a vagal response, leading to cardiac arrhythmias such as bradycardia.

Other complications could include: vomiting, if the patient has a sensitive gag reflex; mucosal damage creating bleeding; or even atelectasis.

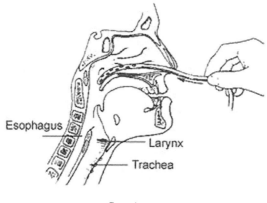

Suction

Sometimes, despite all we do, our patient still will continue to decline and will require either non-invasive ventilation or intubation.

A good candidate for non-invasive ventilation is a patient who is in some form of respiratory distress (tachypnea, hypoxia, hypercarbia, or dyspnea) but is still able to maintain their own airway.

If the patient has an altered level of consciousness, can't protect their airway, or has agonal respirations, they should not be placed on non-invasive ventilation. This patient should be intubated.

NON-INVASIVE VENTILATION: involves using positive pressure to assist the breathing of a non-intubated patient. The two most common forms of non-invasive ventilation are: Continuous Positive Airway Pressure (CPAP) and Bilevel Positive Airway Pressure (BiPAP). I will discuss these modes in more detail in Chapter 8.

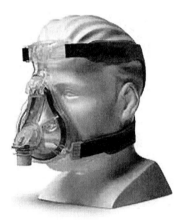

Face Mask

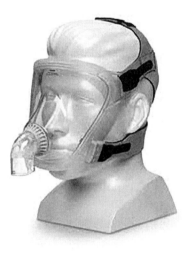

Full Face Mask

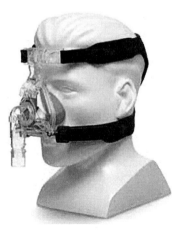

Nasal Mask

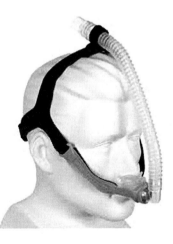

Nasal Pillows

Non-invasive ventilation is administered via a face mask, a nasal mask, nasal pillows, or a full face mask. The mask used will vary from facility to facility, based on what is stocked. It will then be based on the comfort and need of the patient.

The largest complication while using non-invasive ventilation is the mask itself. Comfort is a key component: the patient may feel claustrophobic; they might complain that it fits too tight, or they might say that it is too hot. Skin breakdown is another common problem since the masks are fit rather tightly in order to create enough of an airtight seal for the positive pressure to be effective. The most common breakdown happens at the bridge of the nose. In cases such as these, the nasal pillows or full face mask may be good alternatives.

The positive airflow presents the next largest set of complications. Unless it is humidified adequately, the nasal passages may dry out and lower airway secretions may become thicker and harder to expectorate. This high airflow can also cause gastric distension, eye irritation, and ear pain.

Intubation

If all options up to this point have failed, or if the options mentioned above are not appropriate for your patient, then the final step would be intubation.

INTUBATION: is the process of placing an artificial airway, or an endotracheal tube, into the trachea for the purpose of positive pressure ventilation and/or secretion removal.

An endotracheal tube (ETT) is inserted either orally or nasally with the most common method being orally. It is then secured to the patient's head with tape, tie, or a commercial ETT holder. At the distal end of the tube is a balloon; it is inflated by inserting a 10 cc syringe into the pilot balloon located at the proximal end of the tube. The purpose of the balloon is to create an airtight seal, so the air we are trying to place into the lungs stays in the lungs and does not leak out around the ETT. Just enough air is placed in the balloon to prevent an air leak. If too much air is placed in the balloon, it might exert too much pressure against the tracheal wall, thus occluding blood flow. The long-term effect of this could lead to a tracheal necrosis and stenosis.

The biggest problem that I have seen when it comes to the intubation process is "panic." Even if it is an emergency situation, the best advice I can give is to "stay calm!" When any member of the intubation party panics, it creates a more stressful situation for everyone else, which usually leads to more errors.

I am not going to go into the entire procedure for intubation, but I will cover the equipment necessary to perform the task. Usually, the nurse or respiratory therapist will gather the equipment.

Intubation equipment:

1. Endotracheal Tube (There are various sizes of ETTs. Ask the physician what size they would like. For the adult population, a 7.5 mm or 8.0 mm is common.)

   a. Before handing over the ETT, inflate the balloon to make sure it is patent. If it is, deflate the balloon but leave the 10 cc syringe attached, so it is ready to be inflated after intubation.

2. 10 cc Syringe (as noted above)

3. Stylet (This is a rigid wire that inserts into the ETT. The stylet allows the flexible ETT to be stiffer, thus making intubation easier. When inserting the stylet, make sure it does not extend beyond the distal end of the ETT; if this happens, it could cause a tracheal tear. Bend the proximal end of the stylet so it stays in place within the ETT.)

4. Laryngoscope Blade (There are two types of blades in various sizes that can be used. The miller blades are

straight, while the mac blades are curved. The one used is typically the physician's preference, so just ask what they want. Both blades have a light bulb in them. Make sure the light bulb is secure and won't come loose during the procedure.)

5. Laryngoscope Handle (This is the power source for the laryngoscope blade. Attach the blade to the handle, and the light should automatically come on. If it does not, change the batteries in the handle and/or the bulb in the blade. There should always be spare batteries and bulbs in every intubation kit.)

6. Oropharyngeal Airway (This can be used as a bite block or used for a more stable airway while performing bag mask ventilation prior to intubation.)

7. Ambu Bag with PEEP Valve (Used to provide bag mask ventilation prior to intubation and also to provide bag/tube ventilation after intubation and before placing on the ventilator. Always be sure that there is an Ambu bag with a mask and a PEEP valve at the bedside of every intubated patient. This is necessary should the patient become accidentally extubated.)

8. Tape, Tie, or use a Commercial ETT Holding Device (Whatever your facility uses to secure the ETT in place after intubation.)

9. Stethoscope (To listen to the lungs after intubation, insuring proper tube placement.)

10. End Tidal CO_2 Detector (This is an adaptor that connects between the ETT and the Ambu bag after intubation. The filter in this device is usually the color purple; CO_2 leaving the patient's lungs will change this color to yellow. This color change is one way to confirm that the ETT is in the correct position.)

11. Suction Device with Yankauer (To clear away any secretions that might be in the oral cavity, which prevent the

person doing the intubation from visualizing the vocal cords where the ETT must pass to enter the trachea.)

Your facility may require you to have other equipment present, but this is the most common equipment required at any facility.

Once the ETT is in place, you need to make sure it is secured and in the right place. The way to determine if it is in the right place has been mentioned above; however, here are all the ways used to confirm ETT placement:

- Direct visualization of the ETT passing through the vocal cords
- Color change from the CO_2 detector
- Equal bilateral breath sounds from the lungs
- Absence of gastric sounds over the stomach during inspiration
- Visualization via chest x-ray

Along the side of the ETT are numbers marking how far the tube is advanced into the airway. Once the ETT placement is confirmed, note the marking. The number you want to record will be the number at the level of the lip or gum. I prefer the gum as the lips can swell and alter the reading of the location.

The other type of airway you will commonly see in your patient is a tracheostomy tube. This tube is surgically placed directly into the trachea through the anterior portion of the neck. Since the tracheostomy does not have to bypass the upper airways, it is much shorter than an ETT.

Whether your patient has an ETT or an endotracheal tube, your job of airway management has just begun. Once an artificial airway is in place, you must insure that it stays that way. Make sure to regularly check that the device securing the tube is still holding it securely. Throughout your shift, see that the placement of the tube is marked at the same position as was noted

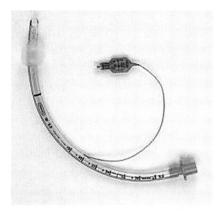

Endotracheal Tube

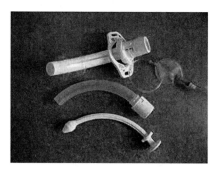

Tracheostomy Tube

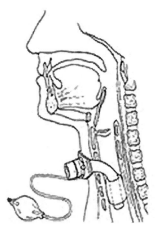

Trach Tube Insertion

after tube confirmation was made. Anytime the patient is being moved, assign one person to hold onto and/or monitor the tube to prevent accidental dislodgement.

Suctioning can also be performed via an endotracheal tube or tracheostomy tube. It can be performed via an open circuit technique or closed circuit technique. The closed circuit technique is preferable because the patient never becomes disconnected from the ventilator. This is vital for infection control purposes and to prevent lung "derecruitment."

Open Circuit Suction Technique:

1. Wash hands and don personal protective equipment: protective eyewear, mask, gloves, and gown (if indicated).
2. Turn on the suction regulator and adjust it between -80 to -120 mm Hg for adults and -60 to -80 mm Hg for pediatrics.
3. Open the suction catheter and connect it to the suction regulator while maintaining its sterile integrity.
4. Connect the Ambu bag to an oxygen flow meter and turn the flow up all the way.
5. Don sterile gloves.
6. Have a second therapist and/or nurse disconnect the patient from the ventilator and connect the Ambu bag. Provide at least one minute of manual respirations to hyperoxygenate the patient.
7. Remove the suction catheter while maintaining its sterile integrity.
8. Have the other therapist disconnect the Ambu bag from the ETT.
9. Insert the catheter without applying suction until you hit resistance; this is usually the carina.
10. Slowly withdraw the suction catheter while applying suction.
11. Take no more than 10 to 15 seconds for suctioning.
12. If no more suctioning is needed, reconnect the patient to the ventilator.
13. If more suctioning is required, reconnect to the Ambu bag to preoxygenate the patient.

Well, no medical technique can occur without debate and controversy, and suctioning is no different.

It is suggested that you can instill 5 to 10 ml of normal saline into the ETT to "loosen" secretions. There are, however, studies that claim that this has no benefit, and more secretions are not removed by doing this technique. They go on further to suggest that by doing this, you could actually cause more harm than good. I have read reports that dispute this claim and state the studies are inconclusive.

Speaking from experience, I have personally seen better results with a normal saline "lavage." This is also common practice for a procedure known as a "bronchoscopy," where they instill far greater amounts than 5 to 10 ml. The facility in which you work may have a specific policy regarding this topic, so please be sure to look it up and follow the recommended practice.

The next controversial topic is that of how you should apply suction. Some literature recommends intermittent suction, while others indicate continuous suction.

The case for intermittent suction is that it minimizes the risk of the damage that the suction can cause to the airways.

The advocates for continuous suction state that there has been no "evidence" of damage from suction, and that every time you interrupt the flow of the suction, you minimize the effectiveness of the suctioning procedure.

I use continuous suction and always have. After 17 years, I can honestly say I have not once seen damage as a result from continuous suction. But as in the case of "lavage or no lavage," your facility might have a particular policy regarding this issue. Always follow the policy and procedure established by your employer.

CLOSED CIRCUIT SUCTION: involves the use of a multiple use tracheal suction catheter, which is incorporated into the ventilator circuit via a standard T-piece elbow or double swivel elbow. This allows for the continuation of mechanical ventilation during suctioning, reducing the potential for infection and derecruitment associated with the disconnection of the patient from the ventilator.

Closed circuit suction technique:

1. Wash hands and don personal protective equipment.
2. Turn on the suction regulator and adjust it between -80 to -120 mm Hg for adults and -60 to -80 mm Hg for pediatrics.
3. Pre-oxygenate the patient with 100% oxygen.
4. Unlock the protective-locking mechanism to allow for suction.
5. Insert the suction catheter until resistance is met.
6. Apply suction and slowly remove the catheter.
7. Re-oxygenate if more suctioning is required.

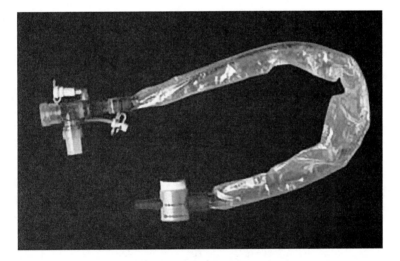

Closed System Suction Catheter

Extubation

I know, I haven't even talked about the modes of ventilation, and I'm already discussing extubation. I hate to put the cart before the horse, but I see the extubation procedure as an airway management issue. There are a variety of criteria involved in making the decision to extubate the patient. The criteria I wish to cover pertain to the ability of the patient to maintain their own airway.

Some of the key functions you will want to assess the patient for would be: mentation, ability to follow commands, ability to cough effectively, and sedation control.

A function that is normally done by the respiratory therapist is a test to see if there is a "cuff leak." Remember earlier I mentioned that there is a balloon at the end of the endotracheal tube that inflates and maintains a sealed airway. The therapist will deflate the cuff and listen for sounds of air escaping around the tube. If no air is heard, it could be an indication that there is some airway swelling present, and it could be risky to extubate the patient at this time.

Extubating a patient with airway edema could result in the airway completely swelling shut after extubation. This would make it virtually impossible to re-intubate the patient and may result in an emergency cricothyroidotomy.

Once it has been determined that the patient is ready to be extubated, you will want to make sure you have all the equipment needed:

- Suction regulator
- Yankauer
- 10 cc syringe
- Towel
- Some type of supplemental oxygen device

Other equipment you may want to have:

- Ambu bag with mask and PEEP valve (in case things don't go well)
- Intubation kit (again, in case the patient fails and needs to be re-intubated quickly)
- Cricothyroidotomoy kit

- Racemic epinephrine for nebulization
- Cool mist aerosol

Steps in Extubation:

- Don protective equipment.
- Explain the procedure to the patient.
- Suction the ETT tube prior to extubation.
- Unsecure the ETT from the patient.
- Suction out the mouth.
- Instruct the patient to cough at the count of three when you pull the tube out.
- Deflate the cuff.
- Count to three and remove the tube.

After extubation, you should immediately assess the patient for any signs of distress. Monitor the oxygen saturation, the work of breathing, the respiratory rate, the heart rate, and breath sounds. Also assess the patient's level of orientation, ability to cough, and subjective symptoms.

Failure of extubation primarily is limited to two different reasons:

1) The patient simply cannot protect their airway or breathe effectively.
2) Airway edema is created and puts the stability of the airway at risk.

The way to determine airway edema is primarily through breath sounds. A high-pitched stridor can be heard when the airway swelling increases. Use of racemic epinephrine nebulizers or cool mist aerosols might alleviate this problem. If not, re-intubation is likely.

It is common for the throat to be sore and the voice to be hoarse after extubation. Having an ETT resting against the vocal cords can cause irritation. Inform the patient that they might experience this and that it is normal and will go away.

7

Introduction to Mechanical Ventilation

History

Respiratory and mechanical ventilation are perhaps the most important aspects of patient care existing today. In ACLS and BLS, the ABCs are drilled into your mind. Respiratory is two-thirds of the ABCs (airway and breathing). Even in the Bible, the significance of the airway is discussed. Genesis 2:7 (KJV) states, "And the Lord God formed man of the dust of the ground and breathed into his nostrils the breath of life, and man became a living soul." So when you really think about it, the respiratory profession is the oldest recorded.

Paracelsus (1493 – 1541) is credited with creating the first form of mechanical ventilation when he placed a tube into a patient's mouth and ventilated the patient with fireplace bellows.

Andreas Vesalius (1514 – 1564) was the first person to have placed a reed or cannula into the trachea of an animal and blow into it.

Robert Hooke (1635 – 1703) was a member of a prominent academic group, The Royal Society, in London. In this group,

84

Hooke was involved in many experiments, including the use of bellows to keep an animal alive while the thorax was opened.

In 1767, the Dutch formed the Society for the Rescue of Drowned Persons. Their most notable contributions included the use of mouth-to-mouth resuscitation as well as chest compressions.

In 1871, Friedrich Trendelenburg, a surgeon, introduced the first cuffed tube used in preventing aspiration during surgery of the larynx.

In 1911, Dräger developed the pulmotor, an artificial breathing device used by fire and police units for resuscitation.

The polio epidemic of the 1950s brought on the rapid advancement of negative pressure ventilation. Although forms of it have been in existence since the mid-1800s, it took a medical crisis to put urgency on the matter. Negative pressure ventilation, most commonly found in "the iron lung," was a process in which a patient was placed in a chamber that covered the chest and abdomen. The chamber would allow ventilation to occur through the creating of a negative pressure outside of the chest. This negative pressure would transfer through to the thoracic cavity, causing air to move into the lungs. The biggest drawback of this form of ventilation was that there was no access to the patient's chest for a physical exam.

Positive pressure ventilation, as described earlier through the works of Paracelsus, has been slowly developing throughout history and is the primary method used to ventilate today. It is for this reason that the remainder of this text discusses the modes of positive pressure ventilation.

Definitions

The world of medicine has a language all its own. We have medical terms, lingo, and abbreviations that may have some outsiders believing that they have entered into a foreign country.

Mechanical ventilation is no different. Sometimes when we teach about mechanical ventilation, we overload our students with definitions and abbreviations so much so that it hampers their ability to grasp the basics. Before I get started, you will need to understand and become familiar with the "basic" definitions and abbreviations used in the following chapters.

BAROTRAUMA: Damage to the lungs caused by high pressure or high volume.

COMPLIANCE (C_L): A measurement of the lungs' ability to expand.

F_1O_2: The percentage of oxygen delivered to the patient.

MINUTE VENTILATION: The amount of air breathed in and out in one minute. This is calculated as respiratory rate X tidal volume.

PEAK INSPIRATORY PRESSURE (PIP): The highest pressure measured in the lungs upon inspiration.

POSITIVE END EXPIRATORY PRESSURE (PEEP): A maneuver that maintains the patient's airway pressure above baseline. PEEP helps to maintain recruited alveoli and is measured in cm H_2O.

PLATEAU PRESSURE (P PL): The measurement of pressure applied to the small airways and alveoli during inspiration. Plateau pressure is measured during a period when no gas flow is entering the lungs (a static condition). This is done by adding an inspiratory pause of 0.5 to 1 second after peak inspiratory pressure is achieved. This pressure can also reflect how easily the alveoli can be distended.

PNEUMOTHORAX: A hole in the lungs which leads to air or gas entering into the pleural space of the thorax. This condition can lead to lung collapse.

PRESSURE SUPPORT: An amount of pressure measured in cm H_2O delivered to a patient during a spontaneous inspiration.

RESPIRATORY RATE (R.R. OR BREATHS/MINUTE): The number of breaths a person takes or receives from the ventilator in one minute.

TIDAL VOLUME (V_T): The amount of air breathed in or out during a single breath.

Anatomy and Physiology

The Respiratory Cycle:

To understand how best to use a ventilator, you must first understand some basic principles about how you breathe.

Air moves from an area of high pressure to an area of low pressure. This difference in pressure is called a pressure gradient. Therefore, to have air outside of the body move into the lungs, a pressure gradient must occur. This pressure gradient is caused by thoracic expansion and contraction.

We often think of breathing as just an in-and-out phase when, in fact, there are four phases of the respiratory cycle.

Phase 1: Beginning of inspiration:

The respiratory muscles begin to contract, causing the thorax to expand. This process creates a negative pressure in the airways, and air begins to enter the lungs.

Phase 2: End inspiration:

The respiratory muscles have stopped contracting during this phase. As the atmospheric pressure equilibrates with the lung pressure, inspiration stops.

Phase 3: Beginning of exhalation:

As the respiratory muscles relax, the pressure in the lungs becomes greater than the atmospheric pressure. At this point, air exits the lungs back into the atmosphere.

Phase 4: End exhalation:

The pressure in the lungs is equal to the atmospheric pressure (the air pressure that exists outside of the body). Air does not move either into or out of the lungs during this phase.

Now that you have an understanding of the ventilation phases, I will describe how mechanical ventilation plays a role during each phase.

Phase 1: Beginning of inhalation:

In mechanical ventilation, this phase is called the triggering mechanism. There are four ways in which the ventilator can be triggered to begin inspiration: pressure, flow, time, or volume.

PRESSURE-TRIGGERED: ventilation came about when it was determined that patients may want to take a spontaneous breath, which is also known as assisted ventilation. The operator sets the pressure sensitivity on the ventilator. As the patient attempts to take a breath, they create a negative pressure against the circuit. When the set pressure is reached, the ventilator will begin the breath.

FLOW-TRIGGERED: inspiration requires a ventilator that has the ability to sense inspiratory flow from the patient. Many old style ventilators do not have this capability. For the newer ones that do have this feature, the inspiration begins when the ventilator senses a drop in the circuit flow, which is caused by the spontaneous inspiratory effort from the patient.

TIME-TRIGGERED: ventilation is also called controlled ventilation. In this mode, the patient cannot cycle a breath. The ventilator/operator sets or controls the respiratory rate. If the rate is set at 12 times per minute, then the ventilator will cycle a breath every 5 seconds.

VOLUME-TRIGGERED: inspiration from the ventilator begins when a preset volume is reached on a spontaneous effort from the patient.

Phase 2: End Inspiration:

This phase is also known as the cycling method. As in the beginning of inspiration, the ending of inspiration can be pressure-cycled, flow-cycled, time-cycled, or volume-cycled.

PRESSURE-CYCLED: Inspiration will stop when a preset pressure is reached within the patient circuit. The tidal volume that the patient will receive will be variable. It will change based on the patient's compliance, inspiratory time, and flow pattern. In cases where a larger circuit leak is present, the preset pressure may never be reached. Therefore, the inspiratory phase will not stop, and the patient will not receive an adequate tidal volume.

TIME-CYCLED: This cycle occurs when you are able to set the inspiratory time on the ventilator. When the inspiratory phase reaches this set time, the ventilator will begin the expiratory phase. In time-cycled ventilation, the flow, tidal volume, and pressure will be variable. If you have a set tidal volume, as in volume control ventilation, with a set inspiratory time of one second, then the ventilator needs to push this amount of air into the lungs during this set time. The higher the tidal volume, the greater the flow of gas will need to be to reach the goal. The peak inspiratory pressure will also be limited. It will take a greater amount of pressure to push the air into the lungs if the inspiratory time is not long enough. If you have a set pressure to achieve rather than a tidal volume, then the volume the patient will receive is going to be variable. If you have the set pressure at 20 cm H_2O with an inspiratory time of one second, you will give the patient a greater tidal volume than if the inspiratory time was only .75 seconds.

VOLUME-CYCLED: Inspiration will stop when a preset volume is reached. The inspiratory pressure will be variable and is primarily dependent on the patient's lung condition. If the lungs are stiff or non-compliant, it will take a greater amount of pressure to deliver the volume than on a patient with healthy lungs, which are easily expandable.

PHASES 3 AND 4: End of Exhalation and Beginning of Inspiratory Phase

I will combine these two phases into what is called the expiratory phase. During the exhalation phase, air moves out of the lungs and returns to the expiratory side of the ventilator. Most of the newer ventilators on the market today possess microchip technology, which provides the ability to measure the volumes returned from the patient. It is important to measure the exhaled volumes to see if they match the inspired volumes. If the volume coming back from the patient is less than what was delivered, then you need to diagnose the problem. Some of the most common problems are:

- Circuit disconnect on the expiratory side
- Expiratory time is not long enough, creating air trapping or auto PEEP
- Expiratory filters may be saturated with moisture, therefore not allowing the flow of air to pass through to the ventilator

During the exhalation phase, the weight of the chest and the natural tendency of the respiratory muscles to relax will allow for the exhalation to occur. The pressure gradient that now exists between the lungs and the atmospheric air will also play a factor in the exhalation process. When mechanically ventilating a patient, the primary factor for stopping exhalation is time. Most modes of ventilation have a set respiratory rate with a set inspiratory time, thus automatically setting the expiratory time. For example, if you have a set respiratory rate of 12 breaths per minute with a one second inspiratory time, then you will have a 4 second expiratory time.

60 seconds ÷ 12 bpm = 5 seconds
5 seconds – 1 second inspiratory time = 4 seconds expiratory time

In modes where there is no set respiratory rate, such as pressure support or volume support, the patient will spontaneously begin the next inspiratory cycle, thus ending the expiratory phase.

PEEP is another factor that affects the expiratory phase. PEEP (Positive End Expiratory Pressure) is a set amount of pressure existing in the ventilator circuit during the exhalation phase. This pressure transfers from the circuit to the patient's airways and will keep the alveoli somewhat distended during exhalation. PEEP prevents partial or complete collapse of the airways during exhalation, thus creating a greater inspiratory pressure to open these airways. Again, if there is not enough time for a patient to fully exhale before the next breath begins, air trapping or auto PEEP may occur. The air that did not have time to exit the lungs remains and creates its own amount of pressure against the alveoli. This pressure is called auto PEEP and will not allow the alveoli to collapse completely.

Since you have determined that PEEP can be good, you may be asking what is so bad about auto PEEP? PEEP and auto

PEEP need to be managed carefully. There can be detrimental effects to having excessive PEEP. Primarily, too much PEEP can transfer this pressure against the vessels of the heart and can lead to a decreased blood pressure. It is very important to monitor the patient's blood pressure when administering PEEP.

Resistance

Airway resistance is the impedance or opposition to the flow of gas. The airway resistance equation is:

$$R = \frac{\Delta P}{v} = \frac{Patm - Pa}{v}$$

R = Resistance
ΔP = Change in Pressure
V = Volume
Patm = Atmospheric Pressure
Pa = Alveolar Pressure

Normal airway resistance is 0.6 to 2.4 cm H_2O/L/Sec.

We must discuss the two types of flow in order to fully understand all aspects of airway resistance: laminar flow and turbulent flow. Water flowing through a pipe is experiencing laminar flow, while water flowing through a rocky riverbed is experiencing turbulent flow. The same principle applies to your airways.

Reynolds number is an equation developed by Osborne Reynolds, a British engineer and physicist, and is useful in determining if the flow of gas is smooth (laminar) or rough (turbulent).

Reynolds number: $N_R = \dfrac{v \times d \times 2r}{\eta}$

v = Velocity
d = Density
r = Radius
η = Viscosity

Reynolds number of < 2000 represents laminar flow, while a number > 2000 represents turbulent flow.

Poiseuille's law describes the physical attributes of laminar flow and puts it into an equation:

$R = 8l\eta/\pi r^4$
R = Resistance
l = Length of Tubing
r = Radius of Tubing

In laminar flow, the radius of the tubing will have a greater effect than any other factor in the above equation. Based on Poiseuille's law, if you double the size of the tubing, or in this case the airway, you will decrease the resistance by a factor of 16, while a decrease in the airway by one-half will cause a 16-fold increase in resistance.

Turbulent flow does not have an equation like that of laminar flow. Go back to the example of water flowing through a rocky riverbed. Various factors affect the flow of the water: the size of the rocks, the number of rocks, other debris that may exist, and living organisms within the water. The human airway is similar to the riverbed when it comes to understanding how turbulent flow works. Flow is affected by the structures of the upper airways, such as the turbinate bones in the nasal passageway or even the hairs of the nose (vibrissae). It may also be affected by: secretions; obstructions, such as aspirated food; and natural bifurcations of the airways. The more obstructions present, the greater the resistance to the flow.

Treating airway resistance is, for the most part, quite simple. In the case of laminar resistance, it is simply a matter of increasing the size of the airway. This can be done by changing the endotracheal tube to a larger size or by the delivery of a bronchodilator to increase the diameter of the anatomical airways. Turbulent resistance may be corrected by: suctioning chest percussion, adding humidification, and the use of heliox (a low-density gas mixture of oxygen and helium).

8

Modes of Mechanical Ventilation

As you are well aware, there are many modes of mechanical ventilation, but I will be covering only the basic modes. Many other advanced modes exist, yet they would require more extensive analysis. My goal is to give you a firm foundation on which to build, and building on a shaky foundation yields an unstable structure as teaching advanced technique before the basics are fully understood yields an unstable education.

I will begin with the modes that provide the most support to the patient and work through to the modes in which the patient is doing most of the work. It is also important to understand that I am teaching the basics of mechanical ventilation. After completing this book, your goal should be to know and understand the following:

- Definitions of basic mechanical ventilation
- Abbreviations used in basic mechanical ventilation
- Modes of basic mechanical ventilation
- Normal blood gas values
- Basic ventilator changes to correct out-of-range blood gas values

Reading and understanding this book is *not* enough knowledge for you to make ventilator changes on your own. You must always follow the clinical practice guidelines established by the facility at which you are employed. Now, let's get started!

Controlled Mechanical Ventilation (CMV)

This mode is rarely used today. When you see the word "control" used in describing a mode of ventilation, it means that *you* are taking control, not the patient. In controlled mechanical ventilation, the ventilator takes total control of the patient's breathing. You will enter a set tidal volume and set respiratory rate. What you set is what the patient receives with every breath. Any effort by the patient to breathe above the set rate will be ignored. An example of typical settings is as follows:

Tidal volume:	500 ml
Respiratory rate:	12 breaths/minute
F_IO_2:	40 %
PEEP:	5 cm H_2O

Your patient will receive a tidal volume of 500 ml, 12 times per minute, for a minute ventilation of 6.0 liters (tidal volume x respiratory rate = minute ventilation). This mode is appropriate if the patient is paralyzed by medications and there is no chance of the patient making any inspiratory effort. If the patient does make an effort, that effort will be ignored by the ventilator, and the patient may begin fighting with the ventilator.

Volume Control

You may have also heard this mode termed *assist-control*. As in controlled mechanical ventilation, you will again set a tidal volume and respiratory rate for your patient. However, this time, when the patient takes a spontaneous breath above the set respiratory rate, they will receive the same tidal volume delivery that was delivered during a controlled breath. An example of typical volume control settings are as follows:

Tidal volume:	500 ml
Respiratory rate:	12 breaths/minute
F_IO_2:	40%
PEEP:	5 cm H_2O

As you can see, the settings are the same as in the CMV mode. Based on these settings, the patient will receive a controlled breath of 500 ml at least 12 times per minute. If the patient is breathing greater than 12 times per minute, then *each additional breath the patient takes will also be controlled.* The ventilator will deliver 500 ml for each of the spontaneous breaths.

The main advantage of volume control is that it guarantees the patient will receive a set tidal volume and respiratory rate. This means the patient will also receive set minimum minute ventilation. One of the disadvantages of this mode is that although we have a guaranteed tidal volume, the peak inspiratory pressure will vary. If the patient's lungs become stiff and less compliant, the peak inspiratory pressure will rise. This can be dangerous to the patient unless you have set the peak inspiratory alarm at a safe level. The peak inspiratory alarm allows the ventilator to terminate the breath if the peak inspiratory pressure delivered to the patient reaches the limit you have set on the alarm. Nevertheless, even causing a single breath at a high peak inspiratory pressure may cause damage to the patient's lungs. An example of this damage may be barotrauma or possibly a pneumothorax.

Pressure Control

"Control" is, again, the key word in this mode. The ventilator is still taking complete control of the patient's breathing. The key difference between pressure control and volume control is simply how the breath will be delivered. In volume control, you set a certain tidal volume to be delivered with each breath as the peak inspiratory pressure varies. In pressure control, you set a peak inspiratory pressure to be delivered with each breath, and the volume will now vary. An example of typical pressure control settings are as follows:

Peak pressure:	24 cm H_2O
Respiratory rate:	12 breaths/minute
F_IO_2:	40%
PEEP:	5 cm H_2O

The patient on these settings will now receive 12 breaths per minute. On each inhalation, the machine will deliver a breath until 24 cm H_2O is achieved. At that time, the inspiration will stop. Depending on the compliance of the lungs, the amount of volume the patient receives will vary. If the patient is 60 years old, overweight, and has a severe case of pneumonia, then 24 cm H_2O will deliver a far smaller tidal volume than a patient who is 20 years old, has never smoked, and runs two miles every day.

The main advantage of pressure control is safety. It does not matter how poor the compliance of the lungs becomes since each breath will always terminate at the set peak inspiratory pressure. The chance of barotrauma occurring is far less than in volume control. A drawback to pressure control is that it does require more careful monitoring of the patient because, as lung compliance changes, so will the returned tidal volume. Therefore, there is no guaranteed tidal volume or minute ventilation. As lung compliance changes, the respiratory therapist must adjust the set peak pressure in order to keep up with the new demands of the patient. If these changes are not carefully watched, the patient could easily become either over ventilated or under ventilated.

An example of how a patient can be affected by each mode of ventilation might help to explain the differences further. Let us say a patient is rolled onto their side while the nurse is changing the linens. While the patient is rolled over, a mucus plug occludes the left lung. All you are ventilating now is the right lung. In the volume control setting that was previously illustrated, the right lung will now receive the entire tidal volume of 500 ml. This high volume will create a high peak inspiratory pressure, and in just one breath you may have caused significant damage to the airways. Using the same illustration, the patient in pressure control will receive the same peak inspiratory pressure of 24 cm H_2O to the right lung, which is the same amount of pressure delivered before. The patient might be under ventilated until the plug is removed. However, a patient can go quite some time being under ventilated before any harm can occur, while just one breath set at too high of a pressure can be damaging.

Here is another example: after suctioning a patient, the compliance of the lungs has now increased. For the patient in volume control, this means each delivered breath will still be at a tidal volume of 500 ml, but the peak inspiratory pressure needed to achieve this volume has gone down. For the patient in pressure control, the same peak pressure is still being delivered; however, the tidal volume received by the patient has now increased due to the increased compliance of the lungs.

Pressure-Regulated Volume Control (PRVC)

Notice the word "control" appears again in this mode. PRVC is considered by some to be the best of both worlds, combining volume control and pressure control ventilation. When you put a patient on PRVC, as in volume control, you are going to set a tidal volume and respiratory rate. The first breath the machine delivers will be a volume breath delivering the tidal volume you set. The ventilator will measure the plateau pressure used in delivering the initial volume breath as a pressure-controlled breath. *The ventilator will adjust the amount of pressure to deliver to the patient by measuring returned volumes and automatically adjusting the pressure based on those returns.* The change will be in increments of 3 cm H_2O per breath. The maximum peak pressure that will be delivered will be no more than 5 cm H_2O below the set high-pressure alarm. The basic settings for this mode will be the same as in volume control:

Tidal volume:	500 ml
Respiratory rate:	12 breaths/minute
F_IO_2:	40%
PEEP:	5 cm H_2O

Based on these settings, the first breath delivered will be a volume breath of 500 ml. Let us assume the plateau pressure measured in this breath is 24 cm H_2O. The next breath will now be a pressure-controlled breath delivering a breath at 24 cm H_2O. Now, each breath the patient receives will be a pressure breath above the set rate, and the breath is delivered at the set pressure of 24 cm H_2O.

Going back to the scenario used earlier in which one side of the lungs is plugged using the PRVC mode, the right side will still receive only 24 cm H_2O. The volume returned will more likely be a smaller volume as you are only receiving volume from the right side. The next breath will be delivered at 27 cm H_2O. Each additional breath will increase by 3 cm H_2O until the desired volume is achieved or when you have reached a peak inspiratory pressure of 5 cm H_2O below the set high peak pressure alarm. You still run a risk of inducing barotrauma if the condition is not corrected quickly or if the high-pressure alarm is set too high.

Adaptive Support Ventilation (ASV)

The concept of ASV is based on "the least work of breathing" model by Otis in the 1950s. It is a dual-controlled mode that switches from a control type of mode to a SIMV or pressure support type of mode based on the patient's status.

Upon setup, the clinician will input the following information:

- Patient's ideal body weight
- PEEP
- FIO_2
- High-pressure limit alarm
- Percent minute ventilation (% Min. Vol.)

Based on the ideal body weight and the target minute volume, the ventilator will adapt the V_T, rate, pressure, I:E ratio, and mode based on the lung mechanics and pattern of breathing. If the patient is making little to no spontaneous effort, ASV applies volume-targeted pressure control. As the patient starts initiating more spontaneous breaths, ASV transitions from full support to partial support using pressure support breaths. The machine continues to adapt to the changing lung dynamics of the patient throughout all mode changes. Once the patient's tidal volume and respiratory rate meet the goals set, then ASV "backs off" and allows weaning.

Imagine if you set up adaptive support ventilation and enter the following:

IBW	60 kg
PEEP	5 cm H_2O
FIO_2	40%
% Min. Vol.	100%

The ventilator will set a target minute volume of 6.0 liters. The ventilator in this mode sets a target volume of 100 cc/kg/min, thus 100 cc X 60 kg X 1.0 = 6000 cc or 6.0 L/min. If you set the % Min Vol. at 80%, the machine will change the target minute volume to 4.8 L/min (100 cc X 60 kg X .80 = 4800 cc or 4.8 L/min). The range in which you can set the % Min. Vol. is 50 to 350%.

Proportional Assist Ventilation (PAV)

Like pressure support and volume support, proportional assist ventilation is a spontaneous mode of ventilation, so the patient must be spontaneously breathing and have an intact respiratory drive. Basically, this mode works by setting the amount of work or effort you want the ventilator to provide, and the patient provides the rest. The range in which you can select is anywhere from 10 to 90%.

Therefore, if you set it up to 60% proportional assist, the ventilator will provide 60% of the work of breathing while the patient will have to provide the other 40%.

The machine knows how much inspiratory pressure or "effort" it needs to perform by taking constant measurements of the lungs' compliance and resistance. These measurements can change on a breath-to-breath basis, so if the patient is taking in a large breath one moment and a smaller breath the next, the machine automatically compensates for this.

The basic settings are:

- FIO_2 40%
- PEEP   5 cm H_2O
- % Support   80%

Synchronized Intermittent Mandatory Ventilation (SIMV)

This is probably the most commonly used mode in mechanical ventilation today. It is the first mode I discuss where the word "control" does not appear in the title. This means you are relinquishing some of your control and beginning to let the patient take control of her breathing. In other words, you are starting to allow the patient to "wean" off the ventilator.

To understand the concept of weaning, I sometimes compare it to someone who breaks a leg. For a while, the person should not bear weight on that leg. Eventually, they are able to do so. At this point, you do not take the crutches away as the patient is not ready and will most likely fall, potentially causing further harm. Mechanical ventilation is no different. When a patient is finally able to begin breathing on their own, you do not remove all support. You gradually lessen the support of the machine until the patient is ready to be removed from it all together. Sometimes, as in the case of post-op recovery, this process is relatively short. In other cases, such as trauma to the airways, this process can take quite a bit longer.

In SIMV, the fundamental change in the way you deliver mechanical ventilation is with regard to the spontaneous breaths. The first time the patient takes a spontaneous breath, it is no longer a controlled breath but instead a supported breath. A patient with a broken leg who is using crutches and walks without placing any weight on the injured leg is taking a controlled step. When the patient starts applying weight, the crutches are now providing a supported step. When you use this mode of ventilation, you will be using the same settings as previously discussed with the addition of one more setting. The additional setting is called pressure support. I will discuss the basic settings and explain how pressure support works. Here are the basic settings:

Tidal volume:	500 ml
Respiratory rate:	12 breaths/minute
F_IO_2:	40%
PEEP:	5 cm H_2O
Pressure support:	10 cm H_2O

With these settings, the patient will receive 12 breaths per minute with a tidal volume of 500 ml. This time, for each additional breath the patient takes, they will receive 10 cm H_2O of pressure support to help them with their inspiration. Spontaneous tidal volumes will vary depending on patient effort and the amount of pressure support that is set. *The pressure support will cycle on during the spontaneous inhalation cycle only.* It is not present during exhalation or during a machine-controlled breath. As the patient becomes stronger, you will begin to wean the pressure support and the number of machine-cycled breaths delivered to him or her. Some ventilators allow the SIMV mode to be used with volume, pressure, or PRVC to determine the type of machine-cycled breaths.

Pressure Support

In pressure support ventilation, there is no longer a set respiratory rate. All breaths taken are spontaneous breaths; therefore, no machine breaths are required. Each spontaneous breath is aided by the setting on the pressure support. An example of basic settings for pressure support is as follows:

Pressure support:	10 cm H_2O
F_IO_2:	40%
PEEP:	5 cm H_2O

This mode can be used *only* for a spontaneously breathing patient, and, as mentioned above, the pressure support is activated during the inhalation phase. PEEP is the only pressure that remains in the circuit upon exhalation.

Volume Support

Volume support ventilation works a little like PRVC. In volume support, a targeted tidal volume is set. The ventilator automatically adjusts the pressure support needed by the patient to achieve this volume.

Here are the basic settings:

Tidal volume: 500 ml
F_IO_2:   40%
PEEP: 5 cm H_2O

Like in pressure support, this mode can be used *only* for a spontaneously breathing patient.

Continuous Positive Airway Pressure (CPAP)

This mode can be done through invasive or non-invasive measures. An invasive measure means an intubated or trached patient. A non-invasive measure means the ventilation is delivered through a mask, creating a tight seal around the patient's nose and/or mouth. When a pressure is set, this pressure is the same throughout the breathing circuit during the inhalation and exhalation phase. This mode requires the patient to be spontaneously breathing. On most ventilators, CPAP is set with the PEEP button. PEEP is essentially the same as CPAP.

Here are the basic settings:

F_IO_2:   40%
CPAP/PEEP   10 cm H_2O

BiPap

BiPap stands for two levels of positive airway pressure. Technically, it is the same as pressure support ventilation. Two levels of pressure are set: a higher level of pressure during the inhalation phase to augment the patient's spontaneous breathing and a lower level of pressure during the exhalation phase, allowing the patient to exhale easier against a lesser flow. The two settings are typically labeled as IPAP (Inspiratory Positive Airway Pressure) and EPAP (Expiratory Positive Airway Pressure).

Typical settings are as follows:

F_IO_2:   40%
IPAP: 10 cm H_2O
EPAP: 6 cm H_2O

Airway Pressure Release Ventilation (APRV)

APRV is an "open lung strategy" mode of ventilation. This means using a reverse inspiratory to expiratory ratio (I:E) to keep the lungs open for an extended duration followed by a short exhalation time for the purpose of removing CO_2. The patient is able to spontaneously breathe through the entire respiratory cycle.

Another way of looking at this mode is to realize that it is a modified form of CPAP. This mode is not meant for someone who is on paralytics. It is used on the spontaneously breathing patient and provides the added benefit of no paralytics and less sedation for the patient.

You may have also heard this mode called Bi-Vent™ or Bi-Level™, and because of the advanced nature of this mode, I will discuss it in greater detail. You will need to know the basic terminology used with this mode. Some of these terms might vary from ventilator to ventilator, but the meaning is still the same.

P High: The inspiratory pressure (similar to pressure control). It is usually set at 2 to 3 cm of pressure above the mean airway pressure the patient uses on the previous vent setting.

P Low: The same as PEEP, only it is labeled differently. It is the end expiratory pressure set on this mode. It is not used very often and is typically set at zero.

T High: This is basically the inspiratory time or the number of seconds during the inhalation phase. It is normally set at 3 to 4 seconds.

T Low: This is basically the expiratory time or the number of seconds during the exhalation phase. It is normally set at 0.6 to 0.8 seconds initially.

F_IO_2: The O_2 percentage the patient is receiving.

Let us assume these are the settings:

P High: 20 cm H_2O
P Low: 0 cm H_2O
T High: 4 seconds
T Low: 0.7 seconds
F_IO_2:   40%

Based on this information, the patient's lungs will be opened for 4 seconds at the set pressure of 20 cm H_2O. The exhalation phase will last 0.7 seconds before the inhalation phase will start over. The set respiratory rate for the patient in the APRV setting is calculated as such:

60 ÷ (T High + T Low)
60 ÷ (4 + 0.7) = 12.7 breaths/minute

PEEP is not set because you usually allow the patient to create their own intrinsic PEEP or auto PEEP. What is auto PEEP? Auto PEEP is created when the patient is on the mechanical ventilator, and you do not give them enough time to exhale before you start the next inhalation cycle. For example, you deliver a breath of 500 ml to a patient, and the patient is able to exhale only 480 ml before the next breath starts. There is still 20 ml of air in the lungs. This extra air produces a certain amount of pressure against the alveolar wall, creating auto PEEP. In APRV, you have a fairly short exhalation time, which allows the patient to create their own PEEP rather than actually setting the PEEP.

It is important that you always measure the auto PEEP to insure the patient is receiving the correct amount of PEEP. If the auto PEEP is too low, you risk greater pressure against the cardiovascular system, which can result in decreased cardiac output and decreased blood pressure.

I feel the need to discuss this mode in greater detail simply because it is more advanced and takes additional knowledge to operate. Remember, the information I am providing is the basic knowledge needed to understand these modes. *In no way does it qualify you to use these modes unless directed to do so by your employer.* I will now explain the settings used in ARV.

P HIGH: I have already stated this number is usually set at 2 to 3 cm above the mean airway pressure from the previous setting. However, you can "fine tune" this number. If the delivered tidal volume is too low, one option you have to correct it is by increasing P High until the desired tidal volume or minute ventilation is achieved.

PEEP: As I have mentioned earlier, PEEP is usually not indicated in this mode. One exception where PEEP might be acceptable is when the lungs collapse quickly upon exhalation. An example where setting PEEP might be a good idea is when T Low (exhalation time) is set at 0.4 seconds, and the patient still has little or no auto PEEP.

T HIGH: The initial setting, as mentioned before, is usually 3 to 4 seconds. By adjusting T High, either higher or lower, the set respiratory rate will also increase or decrease. By increasing T High, you will decrease the set rate, and by decreasing T High, you will increase the set rate. It is another way to alter the minute ventilation received from the patient. Depending on the I:E ratio, you may have to change T High by as much as 0.5 seconds to see a change in the overall respiratory rate.

T Low: By adjusting T Low, you are adjusting the exhalation time. The normal setting is 0.6 to 0.8 seconds; however, these numbers can vary greatly from patient to patient. One step that must be performed as soon as T Low is set is determining the auto PEEP. Each ventilator has a certain method to use in order to get the calculated auto PEEP. Usually, this consists of an inhalation pause followed quickly by an exhalation pause. Typically, you are shooting for a goal of 5 to 10 cm H_2O. In cases of COPD and other lung diseases, you may see a T Low as long as 1.5 seconds. If you continue to monitor the auto PEEP, then you may continue to increase T Low. You want to be careful, however, that you do not increase it too much and lose the reverse I:E ration, which allows APRV to be so beneficial. Remember, when you adjust T Low, the minute ventilation is also altered.

When T Low is increased, the amount of exhalation time increases, which means more air is exhaled, thus increasing minute ventilation. If you decrease T Low, the minute ventilation is decreased. By changing T Low by just 0.1 second, either up or down, it can create a fairly large change in the minute ventilation. This process is a fairly non-invasive way of altering your volume outcome.

Some ventilators that use this mode allow for the use of pressure support. Most often, pressure support is not needed. During the inspiratory phase of APRV, the lungs are already being held open by the amount of pressure set on P High. The higher this number, the longer the lungs are being held open. When a patient takes a spontaneous breath during the inspiratory phase, they will need only a very small breath to fill the remainder of the lungs. For this reason, the spontaneous tidal volume that is measured by the ventilator is usually a low number. It is common practice to add or increase pressure support when you see a small, spontaneous tidal volume; however, in this case, it is not necessary. In lower P High settings, it may be acceptable to add some pressure support. You must remember that the pressure support set will add to your total peak inspiratory pressure of the patient. The peak inspiratory pressure of a spontaneous breath during the inspiratory phase of APRV is calculated at the sum of P High and pressure support.

The three benefits of using the APRV mode of ventilation are as follows:

1. The longer inspiratory phase allows more time for gas exchange to occur at the alveolar level, thus increasing the PaO_2.
2. The longer inspiratory phase also helps to recruit additional alveoli.
3. The lungs are designed to reabsorb a certain amount of fluid. By holding the lungs open longer, you create a greater surface area, therefore allowing more fluid to be reabsorbed back into the lung tissue. This maneuver is beneficial to the fluid-overloaded patient.

High Frequency Ventilation

High frequency ventilation is considered a "non-conventional" mode of ventilation. As far as the level of understanding, it is an advanced mode, and it can be quite difficult to grasp its concepts. Basically, this mode uses an extremely high respiratory rate with an extremely low tidal volume to achieve ventilation. When in operation, it would appear that you are literally vibrating air into and out of the lungs due to this high rate.

High frequency ventilation should be considered when you have a patient on "conventional" modes of ventilation who is not receiving therapeutic benefits from this modality. In other words, the settings are at 100% F_IO_2, the peak pressure is greater than 30, and the PEEP is as high as you can go without negatively affecting the cardiac output.

The theory behind high frequency ventilation is that gas exchange can occur simply by the flow of air into and out of the lungs, given that the lungs are maintained in an open position. The peak airway pressure is relatively small, at times as low as 10 cm H_2O above baseline; however, with the high rate involved, the mean airway pressure can be comparative to that of "conventional" ventilation. Oxygenation occurs through the process of diffusion, thus the oxygen molecule must be in contact with the cellular wall in order for the process of diffusion to take place. By using a higher rate, there will be more opportunity for the oxygen molecule to have contact, therefore increasing the PAO_2.

Three types of high frequency ventilation exist today: high frequency positive pressure ventilation, high frequency jet ventilation, and high frequency oscillation.

HIGH FREQUENCY POSITIVE PRESSURE VENTILATION: Typically, the respiratory rate in this mode is set for 60 to 100 breaths/min with an I:E ratio of 1:3 or less. Tidal volumes are usually 20 to 30% of those found in traditional ventilation.

HIGH FREQUENCY JET VENTILATION: The respiratory rate is a little higher, ranging from 100 to 200 breaths per minute. The I:E ratio is shortened to a 1:1 ratio, and the peak airway pressure is typically set at 8 to 10 cm H_2O above baseline.

HIGH FREQUENCY OSCILLATION: This mode appears to be a literal vibration of the chest as the respiratory rate dramatically increases from 60 to 3600 breaths per minute (1 to 60 Hertz). Reading about this mode cannot do it justice without actually observing it and witnessing its therapeutic benefits. With such a high respiratory rate, it has been shown that you actually increase the overall mean lung volume without a noticeable change in the mean airway pressure.

Neonatal/Pediatric Ventilation

There are a few considerations that must be kept in mind as you shift your attention towards the care of the neonatal and pediatric population. The most obvious, of course, is the size of your patient. When dealing with such small lungs, your delivery method must be adjusted. There are many methods used when dealing with the ventilation of children. It is not my goal to discuss these methods but to provide you with a little understanding as to what modes are most commonly used and why.

Nasal CPAP is frequently used in the neonatal population. It is a noninvasive way of providing positive pressure through the nose in an attempt to avoid having to intubate the patient. The three most common indications for nasal CPAP are:

1) A spontaneously breathing baby that is in respiratory distress. This is evidenced by nasal flaring, retraction, and grunting.
2) PaO_2 is less than 60 with an F_IO_2 of .60 or greater.
3) When apnea spells are present.

Once the infant is intubated, the most common mode of ventilation would be a mode that is time-cycled and pressure limited, similar to the pressure control modes discussed previously. Time-cycled simply means an inspiratory and expiratory time are set. The machine will cycle each breath based on this time. Pressure limited means a peak inspiratory pressure is set for the machine to deliver. A neonate's lungs are much more delicate than those of an adult, thus you want to be sure not to use an excessively high pressure that could damage the lungs. Since the inspiratory pressure in volume ventilation varies with patient compliance, this mode may not be the best to use in this patient population. Again, in using the pressure limited mode, the minute ventilation will vary. Therefore, a greater amount of attention must be devoted to watching the machine to insure that the patient is never under ventilated based on a change in the compliance of the lungs.

High frequency ventilation is a strategy used more in the infant population rather than the adult population. If the infant is not being oxygenated and/or ventilated appropriately with traditional ventilator modes on high settings, this mode may be an option to consider.

The last strategy to discuss Is Extracorporeal Membrane Oxygenation (ECMO). ECMO is not a mode of ventilation. It is a process that bypasses the lungs. In ECMO the venous blood is removed, usually from the right jugular vein, and sent through a machine that oxygenates the blood through a membrane. The blood is then returned to the body. Bypassing the heart and lungs provides an opportunity for these organs to rest. ECMO is usually reserved for the critically ill child who is in some type of reversible respiratory or cardiac failure.

As the infant grows and enters the pediatric population, the modes of ventilation are basically the same as with the adult population. The respiratory rates and tidal volumes are lower due to the physical nature of the child's lungs. As the child grows and matures, the means of treatment become closer to that of an adult.

Ventilator Alarms

What would the I.C.U. be without alarms? Some people may view alarms as a nuisance that must be endured during a shift; however, as you all know, alarms are an important indication that something is not right. It is vital that you understand ventilator alarms: what they mean, how they should be set, and hot to correct the problem that is being identified. With such a variety of ventilators are on the market, there is a plethora of alarms that exist that you may never encounter. I will cover the most common alarms that everyone should know and be aware of.

HIGH PRESSURE: Measured in cm of H_2O and is usually set at about 10 cm of H_2O above the peak airway pressure that the patient is achieving based on the current ventilator settings. It is important to have this alarm set at the appropriate level. In most ventilators, inspiration will stop once it achieves this value, thus protecting the lungs from dangerously high peak airway pressures that could cause damage such as barotrauma.

Several causes can produce a high peak airway pressure such as: decreased lung compliance, increased secretions, bronchoconstriction, and kinking of the circuit or E.T. Tube. These problems can usually be corrected by suctioning the airway, administering a bronchodialator, or removing the kink from the circuit.

LOW PRESSURE: Measured in cm of H_2O and is usually set at about 10 cm of H_2O below the peak airway pressure that the patient is achieving based on the current ventilator settings. When this alarm sounds, it is most likely an indication the patient has become disconnected from the ventilator or a significant leak has occurred within the circuit. Starting with the patient and working back towards the ventilator, check the entire circuit until you find the leak and/or disconnect and correct the problem. The other possibility is the patient may have become extubated. Remember, when trying to identify a problem, always start with the patient and then proceed to the equipment.

APNEA ALARMS: This alarm may show on the ventilator screen as "BACKUP VENTILATION" and is usually set at 20 seconds. If the patient goes longer than 20 seconds without taking or receiving a breath, the machine will alarm. Most ventilators have backup settings that will activate at this point to ensure the patient is being adequately ventilated. This alarm will usually occur when the patient is in pressure support ventilation and has stopped breathing.

LOW VOLUME: This alarm can either mean low tidal volume or low minute ventilation depending on the ventilator. Either way, it is an indication that the patient is not receiving the volume of air that you would like to achieve. There is no "gold standard" as to where these alarms should be set. For example the minute ventilation alarm is usually set at 2-5 l/min below the minute ventilation that the patient is achieving. The problem is usually patient disconnect from the ventilator or a leak in the ciurcuit. Again, follow the circuit starting at the patient and work your way through until you identify the problem.

HIGH RESPIRATORY RATE: This alarm sounds when the patient is breathing above the value set for the high rate. This problem could be patient discomfort either from pain or ventilator settings. Be sure the patient is adequately sedated or make ventilator changes that would be more comfortable for the patient. Many people ask what changes are appropriate. There is no patent answer to this question. Every patient is different. You will need to test various settings until you find what works best for your patient at that time. Another possible cause could be water in the circuit. If the ventilator is attached to a heated humidifier, water or condensation may form in the tubing. If too much water collects and begins to bubble as air moves through the circuit, the ventilator may misinterpret the bubbling for attempts to breathe by the patient. Simply draining the water from the circuit will correct the problem.

LOW GAS SOURCE: Ventilators are connected to compressed air and oxygen sources either from a tank or piped in through the wall. These sources run at 50 pounds per square inch, which is the pressure needed to run most ventilators. If the ventilator becomes disconnected from the wall, this alarm will sound. Simply reconnect the gas source. If the ventilator is still attached to the gas source, something more serious has occurred. There is a problem with the incoming gas source. The ventilator must be connected to an oxygen tank until maintenance can correct the problem.

Basic Ventilator Changes That Affect Blood Gas Values

In the world of mechanical ventilation, you have the ability to make ventilator changes which can alter the arterial blood gas readings. When looking at blood gas values, the only two you can directly affect are the CO_2 and PaO_2. Indirectly, the HCO_3^- level can also be affected but only as a compensatory mechanism. This leaves you with trying to correct and/or adjust the CO_2 and the PaO_2 levels.

If the PaO_2 levels are low and all of the other values are normal then you have a few options to try and correct this issue. I have listed a few of the more common corrective measures below:

1) Increase the FIO_2: This is usually the most obvious answer; however, given the fact that high levels of oxygen does carry with it a risk to our patient it is not usually the first option I would choose.

2) Increase PEEP: This will hold or "trap" more air in the lungs upon exhalation creating an increased mean airway pressure. Increasing the mean airway pressure increase the opportunity for gas exchange to take place. The biggest risk to high level of PEEP would be that of cardiovascular side effects. Anytime you are making a ventilator change it is essential to monitor the patient's hemodynamic status. If it declines after an adjustment such as an increase in PEEP, then it is quite possible that the higher pressure is impeding the cardiovascular system.

3) Increasing the inspiratory time: By having a higher inspiratory time you are essentially holding the oxygen molecule in the airways for a slightly greater period of time. The more time it is in contact with the alveolar wall, the greater the opportunity for gas exchange to take place.

4) Increase the tidal volume: This can be done in volume modes by simply increasing the set tidal volume, in pressure modes it would be done by increasing the set inspiratory pressure. It is possible that if the tidal volume breath was not large enough than the oxygen may not have been getting far enough into the airway to reach the area of gas exchange.

CO_2 is controlled through the amount of minute ventilation from the patient. Minute ventilation is calculated by multiplying the respiratory rate X the tidal volume. If the CO_2 is too high, then you must increase the minute ventilation to "blow off" more CO_2. If the CO_2 is too low, then the patient is being over ventilated. This can be corrected by decreasing the minute ventilation. Again I have listed a few of the more common corrective measures below:

1) Increase the tidal volume: Done as mentioned above.

2) Increase the respiratory rate

3) Decrease PEEP: If the oxygenation is doing well then decreasing PEEP can help remove CO_2. A decrease in PEEP will allow more air to escape during exhalation.

4) Increasing inspiratory time: Sometimes a high CO_2 level has nothing to do with minute ventilation. I have seen minute ventilations as high as 17 lpm with a resulting high CO_2. That is simply air moving in and out of the lung. If gas exchange is not occurring at the alveolar level then all the air moving and out is not going to help the situation. By having an increased inspiratory time will not only help improve gas exchange for oxygen, but it will also help gas exchange as it relates to carbon dioxide.

No matter what choice you make to attempt and correct the abnormality none of it will do any good if you don't identify what is causing the problem. In fact, the first step should be to identify what is causing the problem. This can help us determine the best course of action to take to treat the patient. Again, the list of abnormalities is extensive. There are volumes of textbooks devoted to this topic alone. Listed next are some of the more common issues:

• The patient may be bronchoconstricted in which case a bronchodilator may help.
• The patient may have a mucus plug thus requiring suctioning.
• The patient may have COPD or other underlying pulmonary condition.
• The patient may have trauma to the lungs such as a pulmonary contusion, multiple rib fractures, hemothorax, or pneumothorax.

- The patient may have developed a serious pulmonary complication known as ARDS (Acute Respiratory Distress Syndrome).
- They may be fluid overloaded creating pulmonary edema.
- They may have a pulmonary embolism.

If you ask 100 different doctors what ventilator changes they would make to improve a patient's status you may not get 100 different answers, but I'm willing to bet you will quite a few different answers. The same goes for what ventilator mode is the best and what is the best way to "wean" someone from the ventilator. My goal here is to get you into the game of understanding where it all comes from. In the end you must do what is commonly accepted practice where you work.

9

Arterial Blood Gases

An arterial blood gas (ABG) is a lab test that produces the following critical information: PaO_2 (oxygen), $PaCO_2$ (carbon dioxide), HCO_3- (bicarbonate), and pH. The blood is drawn from an artery that can measure these values *before* the blood enters the tissues of the body, at which time values can be altered.

When obtaining an arterial blood gas, it is important to insure that you are providing a good sample to the lab. The syringe must be a heparanized syringe to prevent the sample form clotting. The collected sample must be free of air bubbles and quickly delivered to the lab. As soon as the blood is drawn, the values can start changing due to metabolism.

It is essential to understand the basics of arterial blood gas interpretation and to know how ventilator changes can affect the outcome of blood gas. In this section, I will explain what you will need to know in order to have a solid foundation.

As in the mechanical ventilation portion of this book, there are several definitions you will need to learn before continuing:

ACIDEMIA: Occurs when the measured pH is less than 7.35.

ACIDOSIS: A patient condition that causes academia, such as increased CO_2 or decreased HCO_3-.

ALKALEMIA: Occurs when the measured pH in the blood is greater than 7.45.

ALKALOSIS: A patient condition that causes alkalemia, such as decreased CO_2 or increased HCO_3-.

HYPOXEMIA: A PaO_2 that is less than normal in arterial blood.

HYPOXIA: A decreased level of oxygen in the tissues.

HCO_3-: A measurement showing the level of bicarbonate in the blood. Bicarbonate is a buffer found in blood, helping to alter the pH level. This is measured in mEq/L.

PaO_2: The partial pressure of oxygen found in the arterial blood. It is measured in mm Hg.

$PaCO_2$: The partial pressure of carbon dioxide found in the arterial blood. It is measured in mm Hg.

pH: The measure of the acid/base balance found in blood.

NORMAL ABG VALUES	
pH	7.35 – 7.45
$PaCO_2$	35 – 45 mm Hg
HCO_3-	22 – 26 mEq/L
PaO_2	80 – 100 mm Hg

I have not yet discussed the base excess, a value you may see in your blood gas values. The normal value for base excess is -2 to +2, with 0 being ideal. Some institutions use base excess rather than HCO_3-, and there is an ongoing debate over which value is better. For the purpose of this review, rather than writing at length about this debate, I will be using all examples with HCO_3- as my value. Be sure to check with your employer as to which value is being used at your facility.

The Process of ABG Interpretation

Step 1: pH Classification

This is one of the most critical numbers that you should review regarding the blood gas. You must determine if the patient is within normal limits, acidemic, or alkalemic. As previously mentioned, the normal pH is 7.35 to 7.45. If the pH is greater than 7.45, the patient is considered alkalemic. If the pH is less than 7.35, the patient is considered acidemic.

Step 2: $PaCO_2$ Classification

The normal range for $PaCO_2$ is 35 to 45 mm Hg. If the CO_2 is greater than 45, the patient is considered acidotic. If the CO_2 is less than 35, the patient is considered alkalotic. CO_2 affects the pH in an inverse relationship. If the CO_2 increases, the pH will decrease. If the CO_2 decreases, the pH will increase. The pH may also be within normal limits, but remember, you can be acidotic without being acidemic. Acidosis is the condition in which leads to acidemia. The proper terminology for an abnormal CO_2 value is either respiratory alkalosis or respiratory acidosis.

$\uparrow$ ventilation = $\downarrow PaCO_2$

$\downarrow$ ventilation = $\uparrow PaCO_2$

Step 3: HCO₃- Classification

The normal range for HCO_3- is 22 to 26 mEq/L. If the HCO_3- is greater than 26, the patient has an alkalotic condition. If the HCO_3- is less than 22, the patient has an acidotic condition. HCO_3- affects the pH in a direct relationship. If the HCO_3- increases, the pH will also increase. If the HCO_3- decreases, the pH will decrease as well. The proper terminology for an abnormal HCO_3- is either metabolic alkalosis or metabolic acidosis.

Step 4: Determine if the condition is compensated or uncompensated

Our bodies are structured in such a way that if something goes wrong, it will often try to correct the problem. If the body finds itself in an acidotic or alkalotic situation, it will try to compensate through the opposite mechanism that caused the problem. For example, if the problem is related to respiratory, the kidneys will either expel the HCO_3- or retain it in an effort to bring the pH within normal range. If the problem is metabolic-related, the breathing pattern will change in such a way as to either eliminate more CO_2 or retain it in an effort to correct the abnormal pH.

There are three categories in which the patient can belong: uncompensated, partially compensate, or fully compensated.

Uncompensated is a condition in which the pH is abnormal, but the body has made no attempt to correct it. For example, the pH is low and the CO_2 is high indicating a respiratory acidosis. The HCO_3^- is within normal limits; therefore, no compensation by the body is present. Uncompensated conditions usually represent an acute change.

Partially compensated is a condition in which the pH is still abnormal; however, the body has begun to make changes in an attempt to correct the problem. Again, you have a respiratory acidosis; but, this time, when you look at the HCO_3^-, it has risen above the normal range in an attempt to correct the pH.

Fully compensated is a condition in which the pH is within normal limits and both the CO_2 and HCO_3^- are out-of-range. Using respiratory acidosis as an example, the pH is normal, and the CO_2 and HCO_3^- are elevated. The Hco_3^- has increased to a point in which the pH was brought back to a normal level. Fully compensated conditions usually represent a chronic change.

Step 5: Evaluate the PaO_2

The normal range for PaO_2 is 80 – 100 mm Hg. For levels below 80, the patient is considered to be hypoxemic, and additional oxygen may be required. For patients on supplemental oxygen, you may see a value higher than 100. In this case, you can start to wean the level of oxygen they are receiving.

BLOOD GAS EXAMPLES

1. pH   7.41
   $PaCO_2$ 43 mm Hg
   HCO_3^- 24 mEq/L
   PaO_2 88 mm Hg

Interpretation: A normal blood gas.

2. pH   7.32
   $PaCO_2$ 49 mm Hg
   HCO_3^- 25 mEq/L
   PaO_2 84 mm Hg

The pH is low indicating acidemia. The $PaCO_2$ is high indicating acidosis. The HCO_3^- is normal; therefore, no compensation has occurred. The PaO_2 is within normal limits.

Interpretation: Uncompensated respiratory acidosis.

3. pH   7.48
   PaCO$_2$ 32 mm Hg
   HCO$_3^-$ 22 mEq/L
   PaO$_2$ 76 mm Hg

The pH is high indicating alkalemia. The PaCO$_2$ is low indicating alkalosis. The HCO$_3^-$ is normal showing no compensation has occurred. The PaO$_2$ is low indicating the patient is also hypoxemic.

Interpretation: Uncompensated respiratory alkalosis.

4. pH   7.30
   PaCO$_2$ 51 mm Hg
   HCO$_3^-$ 27 mEq/L
   PaO$_2$ 69 mm Hg

The pH is low indicating acidemia. The PaCO$_2$ is high indicating acidosis. The HCO$_3^-$ is also high showing there is some level of compensation. Since the pH is still not within normal limits you only have a partial compensation. The PaO$_2$ is low; therefore, the patient is hypoxemic.

Interpretation: Partially compensated respiratory acidosis.

5. pH   7.49
   PaCO$_2$ 30 mm Hg
   HCO$_3^-$ 19 mEq/L
   PaO$_2$ 74 mm Hg

The pH is high indicating alkalemia. The PaCO$_2$ is low indicating alkalosis. The HCO$_3^-$ is also low showing there is some compensation; however, since the pH is still not within normal limits, it is only a partial compensation. The PaO$_2$ is low; therefore, the patient is hypoxemic.

Interpretation: Partially compensated respiratory alkalosis.

6. pH   7.35
   $PaCO_2$ 50 mm Hg
   HCO_3^- 29 mEq/L
   PaO_2 78 mm Hg

The pH is normal. The $PaCO_2$ is high indicating acidosis. The HCO_3^- is high showing the patient is compensating. Since the pH is within normal limits, you have a fully compensated situation. The PaO_2 is low; therefore, the patient is hypoxemic.

Interpretation: Fully compensated respiratory acidosis.

7. pH   7.45
   $PaCO_2$ mm Hg
   HCO_3^- 20 mEq/L
   PaO_2 75 mm Hg

The pH is normal. The $PaCO_2$ is low indicating alkalosis. The HCO_3^- is also low showing there is compensation occurring. Since the pH is within normal limits, this gas is fully compensated. The PaO_2 is low; therefore, the patient is hypoxemic.

Interpretation: Fully compensated respiratory alkalosis.

8. pH   7.48
   $PaCO_2$ 40 mm Hg
   HCO_3^- 28 mEq/L
   PaO_2 80 mm Hg

The pH is low indicating acidemia. The $PaCO_2$ is normal. The HCO_3^- is low indicating acidosis. The PaO_2 is low; therefore, the patient is hypoxemic.

Interpretation: Uncompensated metabolic acidosis.

9. pH   7.48
   $PaCO_2$ 40 mm Hg
   HCO_3^- 28 mEq/L
   PaO_2 80 mm Hg

The pH is high indicating alkalemia. The $PaCO_2$ is normal. The HCO_3^- is high indicating alkalosis. The PaO_2 is normal.

Interpretation: Uncompensated metabolic alkalosis.

10. pH   7.28
    $PaCO_2$ 32 mm Hg
    HCO_3^- 18 mEq/L
    PaO_2 75 mm Hg

The pH is low indicating acidemia. The $PaCO_2$ is decreased creating an alkalotic situation. The patient is not alkalotic indicating there must be some level of compensation occurring. However, only partial compensation is occurring since the pH is still not within normal limits. The HCO_3^- is low indicating acidosis. The PaO_2 is low; therefore, the patient is hypoxemic.

Interpretation: Partially compensated metabolic acidosis.

11. pH   7.54
    $PaCO_2$ 49 mm Hg
    HCO_3^- 32 mEq/L
    PaO_2 88 mm Hg

The pH is high indicating alkalemia. The $PaCO_2$ is increased which should produce an acidotic condition. The patient is not acidemic; therefore, some level of compensation is occurring. The HCO_3^- is high indicating alkalosis. The PaO_2 is within normal limits.

Interpretation: Partially compensated metabolic alkalosis.

12. pH   7.35
    $PaCO_2$ 30 mm Hg
    HCO_3^- 19 mEq/L
    PaO_2 90 mm Hg

The pH is normal. The $PaCO_2$ is low indicating alkalosis. The HCO_3^- is low indicating acidosis. The PaO_2 is within normal limits.

Interpretation: Fully compensated metabolic acidosis.

13. pH   7.44
    $PaCO_2$ 51 mm Hg
    HCO_3^- 17 mEq/L
    PaO_2 58 mm hg

The pH is normal. The $PaCO_2$ is high indicating acidosis. The HCO_3^- is high indicating alkalosis. The PaO_2 is low; therefore, the patient is hypoxemic.

Interpretation: Fully compensated metabolic alkalosis.

14. pH   7.28
    $PaCO_2$ 56 mm Hg
    HCO_3^- 17 mEq/L
    PaO_2 52 mm Hg

The pH is low indicating acidemia. The $PaCO_2$ is high indicating acidosis. The HCO_3^- is low indicating acidosis. The PaO_2 is low; therefore, the patient is hypoxemic.

Interpretation: Combination of metabolic and respiratory acidosis.

15. pH   7.52
    $PaCO_2$ 32 mm Hg
    HCO_3^- 30 mEq/L
    PaO_2 66 mm Hg

The pH is high indicating alkalemia. The $PaCO_2$ is low indicating alkalosis. The HCO_3^- is high indicating alkalosis. The PaO_2 is low; therefore the patient is hypoxemic.

Interpretation: Combination metabolic and respiratory alkalosis.